Contents

Praise for *The Commercial Break Workout*

"There's no excuse NOT to get up off your seat when Linda Buch and Seth Anne Snider-Copley are around. Both of them can motivate even the most sedentary couch potato. Rather than reaching for the remote next time an ad interrupts your TV program, grab *The Commercial Break Workout* and start squatting, lunging, and pulsing your way to better health."

—Linda Castrone, Features Editor, *The Denver Post*

"This book moves adults off the couch and into an exercise program. It just may be what the doctor ordered."

—Marc A. Rabinoff, Ed.D. Professor, Human Performance, Sport and Leisure Studies, Metropolitan State College of Denver

"*The Commercial Break Workout* offers an innovative approach to promoting the benefits of exercise, and I look forward to 'prescribing' this book for my patients."

—William F. Griffith, M.D., OBGyn

"*The Commercial Break Workout* is the fitness book for those of us with the best of intentions but no time to exercise. Effective and easy-to-use, this book is sure to introduce, or re-introduce, exercise to the busy individuals of modern society."

—Jauna L. Hyer, Former President, Ball Dynamics International

"I take the book with me on trips and work out in my hotel room."

—Laurie Csatlos, Flight Attendant

"I was impressed by the authors' imaginative and unique ideas. The concepts presented may well remove another commonly cited obstacle from the path of those interested in improving their health through physical activity."

—Joseph Quatrochi, Ph.D., Associate Professor, Human Performance, Sport and Leisure Studies, Metropolitan State College of Denver

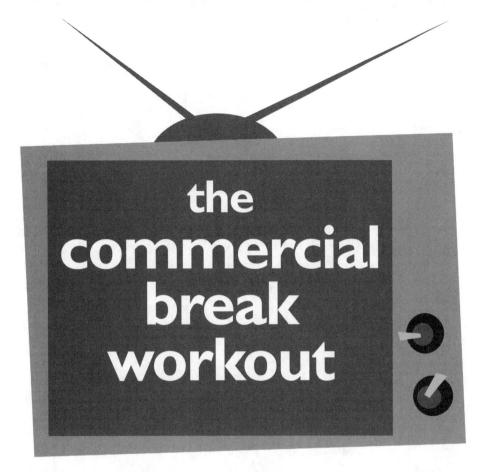

the commercial break workout

Trim and Tone Two Minutes at a Time

Linda J. Buch
Seth Anne Snider-Copley

PRIMA PUBLISHING

Published by Prima Publishing, Roseville, California. Member of the Crown Publishing Group, a division of Random House, Inc.

PRIMA PUBLISHING and colophon are trademarks of Random House, Inc., registered with the United States Patent and Trademark Office.

Design: Knockout Design, Peri Poloni
Illustrations: Bethann Thornburgh

Library of Congress Cataloging-in-Publication Data
   The commercial break workout : trim and tone two minutes at a time / Linda J. Buch, Seth Anne Snider-Copley.
      p.   cm.
   Includes bibliographical references and index.
   ISBN 0-7615-2818-0
   1. Exercise. 2. Physical fitness. I. Snider-Copley, Seth Anne. II. Title.
RA781 .B825   2002
613.7'1—dc21   2002070525

02 03 04 05 BB 10 9 8 7 6 5 4 3 2 1
Printed in the United States of America

First Edition

Visit us online at www.primapublishing.com

To Philo T. Farnsworth, one of the unsung early inventors of the first television, and to RCA's David Sarnoff, whose financial and professional support allowed the final TV product to be completed and perfected. Without these creative folks, this book wouldn't be possible or necessary!

Acknowledgments

We are deeply grateful to Prima Publishing's Denise Sternad for her faith in our work and her vision of what this book needed to become, to Tara Joffe for her invaluable editing skills, and to the rest of the staff at Prima for making this project the fine piece of work it is today. Thanks also go to our agent, Jane Dystel of Jane Dystel Literary Management, for watching our backs. A special thank you to Marc Rabinoff, Ph.D., for his endorsement and support. We extend a very special thanks to Jauna L. Hyer, former president of Ball Dynamics International, for her vision, which helped us to realize ours. We are also grateful to Brian Shearer, Allison Gray, and Susan Bartlett, who all helped keep our vision on track.

Linda J. Buch thanks her parents, Stan and Irene, for their consistent enthusiasm and M. Kay Taylor for her unflagging assistance proofing material at all times of the day and night. Linda Castrone, *Denver Post* editor, has been a wonderful mentor, and I thank her many times over for her support. Also, I could not have done this without the cheerful humor of my fabulous friends, all of my terrific clients, and my cats, Dixie and Bruiser, the world's largest paperweights.

Seth Anne Snider-Copley would like to send a special thanks to Tom Rogers for introducing our idea to Ball Dynamics International, who helped make our dream a reality. Thanks to my husband, Todd Copley, for his everlasting support and enthusiasm during this venture, and a special thanks to my mom, Lynn E. Dodson, for her brainstorming and creativity. More thanks for their ongoing support: Dad (Wayne Snider), grandmother (Lucille Snider), mother-in-law (Dixie Copley), and clients Ernie Panasci and Bob Lees.

introduction

We Have Facts for Your Figures

Go figure . . . American adults seem to be busier than ever. The rigors of juggling work, family, social, and personal obligations make it easy to toss that New Year's resolution of "improving fitness" right into the dumpster. "I cannot squeeze one more thing into my day!" is the familiar refrain. Yet many Americans spend 4 hours of their day sitting and watching television. Oh, the guilt!

Most people think that in order to change their fitness level positively, they have to sweat, groan, work, and then collapse into a huge heap of hurt. If this sounds familiar and has been keeping you sedentary and stretched out on the couch, then *this book is for you!*

Our plan for improving your fitness has no equipment to buy, no special clothing to wear, and, best of all, no schedule changes to your TV-watching plans. *The Commercial Break Workout* will guide you through a series of safe and progressive exercises that you can follow while you enjoy your favorite television programs, while traveling for business or pleasure, or even while you take a break at work. Just minutes at a time will allow you to increase your wellness.

This book includes the primary components of an effective and prudent fitness program:

- posture
- balance
- breathing
- flexibility
- muscle strength
- cardiovascular conditioning

You will perform the stretches and exercises during the commercial breaks of your favorite TV programs. (An average sitcom provides 10 to 12 minutes of commercial break per half-hour.)

As with any exercise program, we recommend that you consult with a physician before you start.

The Facts . . .

According to the Centers for Disease Control and Prevention, more than 500,000 Americans each year suffer from metabolic diseases related to inactivity and a sedentary lifestyle. Billions of dollars are spent annually in the United States on the care and treatment of diseases relating to obesity. Although the term "obesity" may bring to mind images of circus sideshow performers, in reality, if you are 30 percent over your ideal body weight (by medical standards), you are considered obese. More than 61 percent of the American adult population is currently in this category. The number of obese in the United States has doubled in the past twenty years. In the 1990s, diabetes increased by 33 percent among American adults. Coronary heart disease is one of the leading causes of death among Americans today. The common variable is a sedentary lifestyle. Comfortable corpulence comes at a high price: The Centers for Disease Control and Prevention has hypothesized that if all physically inactive Americans became more active, we could save about $117 *billion* in health-care costs.

Congratulations! By buying and using this book, you have taken the first step toward a healthy solution for yourself and for your country.

Your Figure Will Love These Facts and Figures!

The Office of the Surgeon General (C. Everett Koop, M.D.) released the following statement in July 1996: "The Surgeon General has determined that the lack of physical activity is detrimental to your health." In fact, the Surgeon General equated *not* exercising with smoking a pack of cigarettes a day! The Surgeon General's report also stated that health could be improved if "every American [would] accumulate 30 minutes or more of moderate intensity physical activity over the course of most days of the week." This 30 minutes does not have to be all at once. Doing small, short exercise sessions throughout the day *can* improve your health. The old notion of having to do 30 minutes of exercise all at once (or don't bother) has been proven to be misleading. By doing the exercises in *The Commercial Break Workout*, those of you for whom TV watching is a favorite activity can now have your show and watch it, too . . . guilt free!

The Commercial Break Workout begins at a level of light intensity and gradually progresses to a level of moderate intensity. Start off by reading through the book to get familiar with the program. If you haven't worked out in a while, follow the exercises as they are presented in the book. This will ensure that you build up to the proper intensity level without overdoing it.

By using this book, you will positively affect your health, and you won't be thwarted by the frustration and humiliation many people experience at the initial stages of an exercise program. You can begin to enjoy a more healthful and productive lifestyle in the comfort and security of your own home and never miss a single episode of your favorite TV shows.

In the words of Myra J., funny lady on ABC Radio's "Tom Joyner Morning Show," "Get a grip and not a girdle."

Now, tune in to guilt-free TV. . . .

chapter one

Turn Your TV into Your Workout Partner

Another day/week/month/year has passed, and instead of making a trip to the gym, you made a trip to the whine cellar: "I'm too busy, too tired, too fat. What's the use? What good will it do at this point in my life, anyhow? Why bother?" These are vintage whines, are they not? We all have a cache of these stored and ready for use on those days when drowning in self-pity seems to be justified and downright comforting. It's been a hard day. We grab a bag of chips and the remote and head for the couch. The bad news for the TV addict is that inactivity is unhealthy and can potentially increase your chances for premature death or disease. Rather than indulging in self-defeatist sniveling and channel surfing, let's focus on the solution.

According to the Surgeon General's office, 30 minutes of moderate activity per day, during which you expend 150 calories above and beyond what you normally do (a total of 1,050 calories per week), will significantly improve your overall health. You can break up these 30 minutes throughout the day rather than doing them all at once. In fact, by using *The Commercial Break Workout,* you can accomplish your 30-minute goal just by watching 1 hour of television.

Of course, we must mention the fact that there are side effects to all of this activity. Exercising will result in:

1. An increase in energy level

2. A better mood

3. A decrease in blood pressure

4. A decrease in bad cholesterol

5. Better circulation

6. A healthier life

Sounds horrible, doesn't it? Seriously, the best part of a little bit of daily activity is that you can do the stretches and exercises in the comfort of your own home and never miss a favorite TV show. In short, our simple solution can be summarized in one four-letter word: MOVE!

Why Do You Need Muscle?

Your body is made up of fat tissue (the stuff that makes our clothes "shrink") and lean tissue (muscle, bone, organs, and connective tissue). Regular exercise will help you build more lean muscle. A little bit of muscle-building exercise goes a long way because muscle is living tissue that requires anywhere from 35 to 50 calories per pound per day to stay viable. Fat, on the other hand, is just stored energy that can be sustained by only 3 calories per day. A person with a good lean-tissue-to-fat-tissue ratio will burn more calories at rest than will a sedentary person.

Lean tissue contains powerful, furnacelike "engines" called *mitochondria*. Mitochondria produce quick-energy molecules as well as specialized oxidative enzymes that burn fat. The more you stimulate your muscles through strength-training exercises, the more muscle you build. The more muscle you build, the more fuel-burning furnaces your body creates. Keep in mind that muscle is denser than fat. Therefore, a more muscular person can weigh the same as an overfat person and yet look thinner. This is why your weight is far less important than your body's ratio of muscle (lean) tissue to fat tissue.

But what is muscle good for? For starters, strong, healthy muscles will help with all of the following:

• Increase metabolism, which means burning calories in a more efficient manner

• Improve mobility

• Increase structural integrity

Now here is some food for thought: A sedentary person will lose half a pound of muscle per year after age twenty. This means that people who adopt a sedentary lifestyle at age twenty will lose about 15 pounds of lean muscle by the time they reach fifty, even if they maintain the same *weight* as when they were twenty. So just because you may weigh the same, you are not necessarily as lean. Inactivity can also increase the incidence of metabolic diseases, such as diabetes, heart disease, high blood pressure, and osteoporosis.

Getting Started

We recommend that you begin by skimming through the whole book during a commercial break. You may even want to count and time the commercial breaks in one sitcom or hour-long show for yourself. Once you get an idea of how our program works (and see for yourself that there is plenty of time to exercise during the commercials), you can gauge how much physical space you will need to perform the exercises safely. Make sure that your exercise space is in close proximity to your favorite chair or couch and TV, of course!

Once you start the program, go at your own pace. Progress to the next step as you feel comfortable. Begin with one commercial break (about 2 minutes), rest while watching the TV program, and then exercise again during the next set of commercials. Remember, you don't have to do all 30 minutes of exercise at once. For example, say you watch the "Today Show" in the morning before work or "Oprah" during the day, but then you need to stop to pick up the kids, run errands, attend a meeting, and so forth. If that's the case, you can do some of the exercises early in the day and then finish it up from "Jeopardy" through "ER." Or do some of the exercises during "The Sopranos" and the "Evening News"

Tip
To get started, pick two of your favorite shows (on two different days) to be your exercise motivator (not terminator!).

and then finish your program throughout the week during "Frasier," "The West Wing," and "Law and Order."

How to Use This Book

You are never too old, too fat, too tall, too thin, too short, or too out-of-shape (bad hair days don't count either) to begin living a more active life. Believe it or not, the fact that you are relaxing in front of your TV set (perhaps wracked with guilt about not exercising) is a perfect beginning to the most convenient workout program of your life. Let's start with this simple checklist:

- ✔ Are you wearing loose-fitting, comfortable, TV-appropriate clothing?

- ✔ Are you sitting in your favorite couch or chair?

- ✔ Are you watching your favorite TV shows?

- ✔ Do you have a large glass of water?

Did you answer yes to each question? If so, you are ready to begin exercising. Most commercial breaks are about 2½ minutes long, with six to eight different advertisements per break. Each half-hour sitcom can have up to 10 to 12 minutes of commercial time. Therefore, just by exercising during the commercials of a 1-hour program, you can expend 150 or more calories. In a typical evening of TV viewing, you can do 30 to 60 minutes of exercise and lose those unwanted pounds!

Each of the following chapters has specific objectives, such as improving posture, stretching, breathing, muscle strengthening, and cardiovascular (heart/lung) conditioning. Instructions are easy to understand and include plenty of illustrations to demonstrate proper form. The exercises are progressive in their difficulty and intensity. It is important to monitor the intensity of your Commercial Break workouts, especially if exercise is new to you or if you have been away from it for a while. For this reason, we suggest that you start with exercises for improving your posture and balance (chapter 2). You can then move on to the simple stretching techniques that will help improve your flexibility (chapter 3). After that you can get into the strength- and muscle-building aspects of the book (chapters 4, 5, and 6).

DRINK WATER!

Chapter 7 is an introduction to continuous aerobic exercise. The heart is a muscle, too, and it loves a good workout just like the other muscles in your body. Proceed to this chapter at the end of your muscle-strengthening workouts (chapters 4, 5, or 6). The exercises in chapter 7 are intended for use as an introduction to, or as a warm-up for, more extensive cardiovascular activities in which you may eventually wish to participate. The chapter includes some fundamentals concerning blood pressure, cholesterol ("What do all of those numbers mean, anyway?"), and the positive effects of exercise on the cardiorespiratory system (heart and respiration).

If you don't know exactly what exercises you want to do, check out chapter 8. In that chapter, we provide a variety of exercise programs. The programs vary in intensity, from beginner to advanced. To make sure you don't get bored, we include two different options within each level of intensity. Once you get the hang of these programs, get creative and think up some of your own!

In chapter 9, we introduce you to some equipment that you can begin to incorporate into your daily workouts. We rate the equipment in terms of what it can do for your body. The chapter also includes info on where to find the different pieces of equipment.

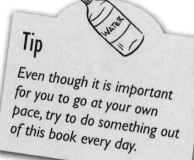

Tip

Even though it is important for you to go at your own pace, try to do something out of this book every day.

Finally, chapter 10 provides basic facts about diet and calories. Enjoying food is not a criminal activity. We want you to enjoy much of what life has to offer; just remember that making educated food choices is a key element to a healthful lifestyle.

Why Water?

Before we get into all of the fun stuff, let's take a second to consider the importance of water, which is the recommended beverage from our checklist. Water is to your body what oil is to your car. Beer is not water. Iced tea is not water. Soda pop is not water. Coffee is not water. Only *water* is water. Water makes up about 60 percent of your body weight and is about 70 percent of your blood volume. The water in your body is where most of the life-sustaining chemical reactions take place. This is why we can live for more than a month without food but only for seven days without water. So, *drink water or die!*

Amazingly, most of us walk around, day in and day out, in a state of partial dehydration. How can you tell if you are becoming dehydrated? "Thirst" would seem like a logical answer. Unfortunately, thirst means that you are already dehydrated. Fortunately, however, it is an early sign. Two other early indicators are fatigue and dark urine with a strong odor. This last sign is one of the best indicators. If your urine is almost clear, you are properly hydrated. Yellow urine indicates the need for more water. More serious signs of dehydration are lightheadedness, inability to concentrate, loss of appetite, heat intolerance, and extreme fatigue.

It is easy to get into the habit of bypassing water. Soft drinks, coffee, fruit juice, sport drinks, alcoholic beverages, and milk are not only popular but also promoted by companies that have extremely large advertising budgets. If you drink these beverages along with—and not instead of—water, then there is less harm. But what is the problem with only drinking beverages other than water? Soft drinks and fruit juices are high in sugar. Caffeine and alcohol are diuretics. Milk has a high concentration of solids in comparison to water. The jury is still out on sport drinks. Some believe that the salt content in sport drinks is too high. Others feel that sport drinks are a distant second to water, and they can, in fact, cause weight-gain. It is generally recommended that sport drinks be consumed in moderation and only when you are participating in endurance sports for longer than 3 hours, which is when your electrolytes (sodium, potassium, and calcium) can become depleted.

Physical activity, even done in front of the TV set, demands that we keep an eye on our fluid intake. Experts say the normal intake should be in ounces what you weigh in kilograms (2.2 kilograms = 1 pound). In other words, a 150-pound person weighs about 68 kilograms (150 ÷ 2.2 = 68). Therefore, 68 ounces of water (eight and a half 8-ounce glasses) would be considered normal consumption. As you become more active, your water consumption should increase. Here are some basic guidelines:

Before exercise: Drink 8–16 ounces of water 2 hours before exercise. Drink another 4–8 ounces immediately prior to exercise.

During exercise: Drink 4–8 ounces every 20 minutes during exercise (during the commercials, in other words).

After exercise: Drink 16 ounces of water for every pound of body weight you have lost.

The fact that water is practically a magic weight-loss potion will probably turn more people into water drinkers than the threat of death by dehydration. According to Dr. Donald S. Robertson of the Southwest Bariatric Nutrition Center, an increase in water intake can actually reduce fat deposits. Here's why: "The kidneys need lots of water to function properly. Without water, the liver takes over. If the liver has to not only do its job of metabolizing stored fat but also do the kidneys' job, it will metabolize less fat. During weight loss the body has a lot more waste to get rid of—like all of that metabolized fat, for example. Water will help flush it away. Retaining water? Drink water. Then, and only then, will the stored water be released. Constipated? Drink water for normal bowel function to return" (www.weight-control.com/doctor.html).

In summary, if you are fatigued, constipated, retaining water, or stuck on a weight-loss plateau, take a look at your water intake.

Onward and forward!! Ladies and gentlemen, start your engines!

chapter two

Posture, Balance, and Breathing

So why is posture so important? Good posture is powerful. It expresses confidence, vitality, and youthfulness. Our bodies are naturally designed to enable us to move gracefully and efficiently, yet many of us fall into poor postural habits. Everyday tensions and stresses are often absorbed by our body and are compounded over time. This has a domino effect throughout the body, creating a structure whose integrity is sorely compromised—emphasis on *sore!* Poor posture is manifested in many different ways. The most common is the "submissive posture" (head down, shoulders rounded); another is the "bully posture" (shoulders shrugged).

11

Spinal misalignments are created when we allow poor posture to persist. It can sometimes even lead to mental and physical problems. Mentally, problems resulting from poor posture can contribute to tension and can heighten stress. Physically, when your spine is compressed, the internal organs are squeezed as if they were in a vise, and lung capacity can decrease, causing your nerves and blood vessels to become constricted. Poor posture also increases the potential for chronic back pain, neck pain, and headaches.

Posture is often a legacy of how we carried ourselves as young children and adolescents. For example, many young girls learn poor posture habits during their formative years, thinking, among other notions, that slouching forward would make them seem shorter or less visible. Similarly, adolescent boys often assume the "bully posture" to look "cool." But you aren't a kid anymore. Stand up tall and pay attention to that annoying little voice in your head telling you, "Stand up straight! Don't slouch!"

Standing and sitting properly will keep your muscles in balance. Balance (symmetry) allows your spinal column and all of the surrounding muscles to work in harmony, thus providing you with increased mobility. Correct alignment carries over into all of your body positions as you move and function throughout the day. Your parents were right—posture is important.

How to Feel Younger and Taller After Just One Commercial Break

Learning to sit and stand correctly will increase structural integrity and will give you a more commanding presence. As a bonus, you will look taller, feel more vital, and have a sound physical foundation to carry you through your day. The illustrations on this page show both "poor" posture and "good" posture when standing.

When you are standing correctly, certain bony landmarks should line up. Notice in the illustration of proper posture how the head is erect and sits directly above the neck and spine? The ears are over the shoulders; the shoulders are over the hipbones; the hipbones bisect the knee joint; and the knee joint bisects the ankle joint.

Throughout this book we remind you to keep your head neutral. A neutral head means that whether you are standing up, sitting down, or doing push-ups, your head should be in alignment with the rest of your body, as shown in the "good posture" illustration.

Posture is important not only while you are standing still. It is important all the time, even when you are carrying the groceries, driving a car, typing a letter, and exercising *while* watching television. Your spinal column and the muscles that surround it work in concert to help ensure painless mobility. Observe yourself right now as you sit watching TV or reading this book. Answer the following questions to assess your posture:

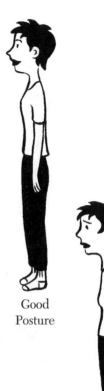

Good
Posture

Poor
Posture

- How are you positioned?

- Is your spine compressed and twisted?

- Do your muscles feel tense and fatigued?

- Are you able to breathe deeply?

Postural awareness is your first step to becoming more mobile and more functional.

Still don't believe us? Try this. Stand in front of the TV and lean to one side as if your body is the minute hand on a clock and your entire body is reaching in a straight line, head to toe, for two o'clock. In the two o'clock position, walk a few steps around the room. Return to the twelve o'clock position and observe how your muscles felt. Did they feel tense and overworked? How did your muscles compensate for this deviant position? Was your breathing more labored? This example may seem extreme, but it should help you see how, over time, poor body position can create one problem after another until your whole body is a zigzagging seesaw of pain and distress.

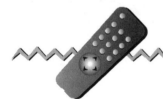
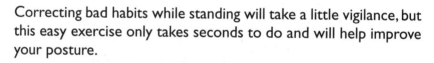

Posture Exercise

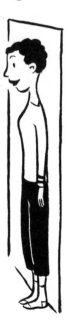

Correcting bad habits while standing will take a little vigilance, but this easy exercise only takes seconds to do and will help improve your posture.

1. If possible, stand against a wall so that the back of your head, shoulder blades, upper part of your butt, and heels all touch the wall. Your arms should hang naturally at your side.

2. Take one step away from the wall.

3. Inhale as you lift your arms away from your sides until they are straight out from your shoulders and parallel to the floor.

4. Turn your arms so that the palms of your hands are facing up to the ceiling.

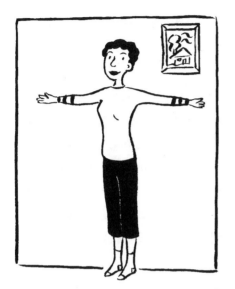 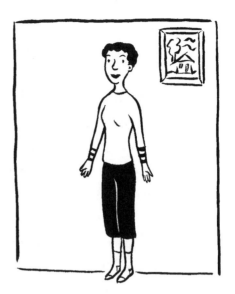

5. Now exhale as you focus on lifting your chest and returning your arms to your side. Keep the palms of your hands facing away from your side.

6. Allow your hands to return to their natural position.

Could you feel how your shoulders pull back and your chest lifts up? If so, then you are on your way to better posture! If not, try it again!

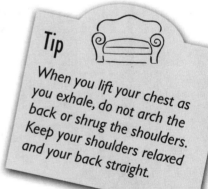

Tip

When you lift your chest as you exhale, do not arch the back or shrug the shoulders. Keep your shoulders relaxed and your back straight.

Why Worry About Balance?

When we are small children learning to walk, we gain balancing skills because we instinctively want to be independent and get moving. Too often, we fall into the habit of sitting at every opportunity, which means balancing skills can be lost. As the saying goes, use it or lose it! As we mature, the issue of balance becomes even more crucial. Many adults are injured unnecessarily because of poor balancing skills.

Perhaps you feel that as long as you can make it up out of a chair to the fridge and back again without falling over, then your balance is just fine. After all, you aren't joining the circus or surfing a big wave, so why worry? But working on your balance is important, even if you are just walking around the house. Good balance fine-tunes the proprioceptors (the sensory-end organs that are sensitive to your body's movements and warn you when you are out of alignment). You don't want to end up face down on the carpet every time you accidentally step on a cat toy or dog bone! So improve your balance to improve your reaction time (which is your response to the signal carried from the brain to the muscle via the proprioceptors).

The good news is that balance is a learned skill that we must use or lose. This means we can do something to improve it. Unless hip replacement surgery is your idea of fun, practice the following exercises to improve your chances of remaining more solidly on your feet.

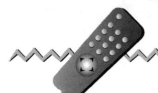

Easy Balance Exercise

Perform this exercise while standing with your shoes off and your feet together.

1. For the first commercial, stand next to a chair. Lift your arms to your side so they are parallel to the floor. Your palms should be facing down to the floor. Close your eyes.

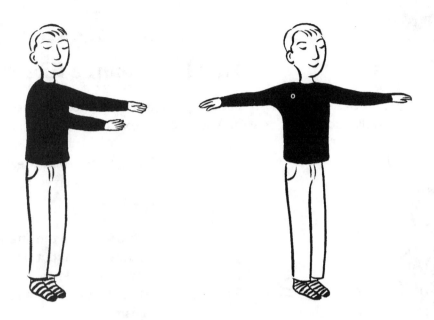

2. Use your muscles and your new posture techniques to keep from wobbling. Stay balanced, breathe normally, and notice which muscles tighten and relax as your body tries to remain stable.

3. Keep your eyes closed as you bring your arms together in front of you, as if you were going to clap your hands. Keep your elbows relaxed.

4. Return your hands to your side.

5. Continue to do this movement throughout the commercial break (no peeking)!

Proceed to the next level only if you've done the Easy Balance Exercise without excessive wobbling or tipping.

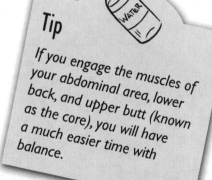

Tip

If you engage the muscles of your abdominal area, lower back, and upper butt (known as the core), you will have a much easier time with balance.

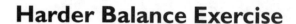

Harder Balance Exercise

Try this exercise, also called the Flamingo, while standing next to a wall, stable chair, or sofa. Again, do this exercise without shoes.

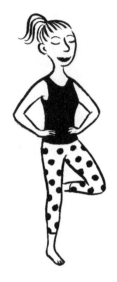

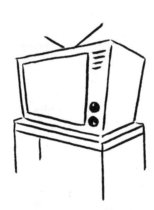

1. Close your eyes. Breathe normally. Keep your knees relaxed.

2. Lift one leg so the lifted foot is beside (but not on) the standing knee. You should look something like a flamingo.

3. Count to 10.

4. Switch to the other foot (still standing like a flamingo). Count to 10 again. Keep those eyes closed!

5. Keep your hips level.

6. Continue to switch legs throughout the entire commercial.

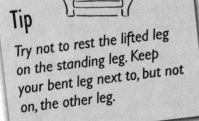

Tip

Try not to rest the lifted leg on the standing leg. Keep your bent leg next to, but not on, the other leg.

Proceed to the next exercise only when you can do the Harder Balance Exercise without excessive wobbling or tipping and without holding onto the wall, chair, or sofa.

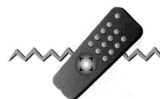

Hardest Balance Exercise

To do this exercise properly, you will need a little walking space. Again, do this without shoes.

1. Stand with your feet together.

2. Close your eyes and take two steps forward.

3. With your eyes still closed, take two steps back.

4. Next take two steps sideways to the right and to the left. Again, no peeking!

Did you feel how your body responded to movement in different directions?

As you do these exercises, pay attention to your breathing. We know (unless you are in training to be an underwater dolphin photographer for "Animal Planet") that you have not been holding your breath this whole time. What kind of breather are you? Are you breathing just from the top of your chest (shallow breather), or are you allowing yourself to breathe all the way down deep into the belly (deep breather)?

The deeper you breathe, the more positively your body will respond to stress, which is one of the contributing factors to coronary heart disease. Unless you are walking behind the exhaust pipe of a bus, or you really are doing underwater photography, breathe deeply . . . just for the health of it!

Breathing Exercises

Let's examine the two kinds of breathing that will be useful with your exercise program.

Relaxed Breathing

1. Lie on your back on the floor and close your eyes. Keep your knees bent with your feet flat on the floor.

2. Place your hands on your lower ribcage and breathe deeply through your nose (inspire). As you inhale, focus on expanding your rib cage and filling your lungs.

3. Hold your breath for a few seconds, then let it out through your mouth (expire).

Suggested Program: Continue this exercise through one commercial break and feel the day's stresses melt away!

Tip

When you inhale, you should feel your fingers separating and your ribcage and lungs expanding like a bellows. When you exhale, you will feel your ribs close.

Active Breathing

Observe your breathing patterns while performing one of the exercises in the book. Are your breaths shallow or deep? Are you holding your breath? When moving, you should always try to breathe deeply from your diaphragm, inhaling at the beginning of the exercise and exhaling during the execution.

As for *heavy* breathing, the only kind we will be addressing is found in chapter 7.

chapter three

Stretching and Flexibility

Stretching is something many people often ignore before turning forty. After age forty, it's something we can hardly live without. But even before turning forty, it is a wonderful thing to do. To keep your body flexible and healthy, it is a good idea to get into the habit of stretching, especially after you exercise.

In this chapter, we show you safe and effective stretches that can easily be done during commercials. Improved flexibility goes hand-in-hand with more resilient muscles and improved mobility, which are real necessities as we mature.

Why Stretch?

Stretching can and should be done every day. It relieves tension, increases blood flow, improves internal organ function, and keeps the muscles supple. Stretching is also a great stress reducer, is often used as a relaxation technique, and when done after a workout, has been found to improve strength. (To learn more about stretching, go to www.fitnessworld.com.)

Flexibility is the ability to move your joints through their full range of motion. Full range of motion is individually determined. Our goal is to help you become more functional in your daily activities. Being able to move your limbs without restriction allows the muscles to receive their necessary nutrients and helps the body remove waste products that can build up in the joints and connective tissue.

Have you ever wondered why a massage feels so good? It's because the massaging of muscles and tissues breaks up the "glue" (waste products), allowing them to move on. This allows nutrients to get to the muscles more efficiently.

Over time, a daily program to improve your flexibility will result in better body alignment, reduced chances for injury, and easier, less painful experiences when doing simple daily activities, such as getting out of a chair, reaching for things on shelves, and even looking over your shoulder while driving or parking a car.

This chapter shows you some basic stretches that we believe you will find helpful and enjoyable.

For most people, the primary benefit to stretching is it makes them feel better. Any argument against stretching can be dismissed by watching a dog or cat. Cats and dogs stretch many times a day and are quintessential examples of relaxation and flexibility! However, don't just jump into stretching. It is always best to stretch when the muscles are warm (after a workout or after a warm bath or shower). Stretching your muscles when "cold" can be like stretching rubber bands that have been in the freezer, and it can cause damage to the very muscles you are trying to help. We recommend, therefore, that you do some walking in place for at least one entire commercial break or do some of the abdominal exercises (chapter 6) before beginning the stretches in this chapter. This will warm the muscles a bit and allow for safer and more productive stretching.

Remember

1. Stretching should feel good. Stretch to a point of resistance, not pain.

2. Stretching is noncompetitive. Do only what feels right for you.

The following stretches can be done either during the commercials of your first half-hour of TV watching or immediately after the corresponding exercises in the chapters to follow. Do each stretch two to three times, holding each for at least 20–30 seconds (about the length of many product commercials).

Neck

Can you look over your shoulder while attempting to parallel park? If not, some neck and shoulder stretches just might be the ticket. Here are three neck exercises designed for both improved flexibility and stress relief.

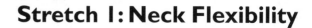

Stretch 1: Neck Flexibility

1. Sit comfortably with proper posture (refer back to chapter 2 for a reminder on proper posture).

2. Exhale while tilting your head forward until your chin touches your chest. Feel the weight of your head stretching the back of your neck.

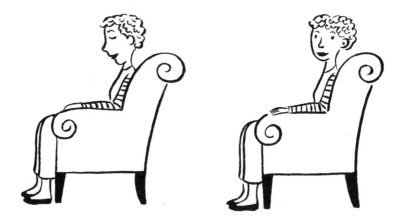

3. Keep your shoulders relaxed. Do not shrug them.

4. Inhale as you return your head to "neutral." Exhale while rotating your head to the left (as if you were trying to look over your left shoulder).

5. Inhale back to center; exhale again as you rotate your head to the right.

6. Continue this entire stretch for one commercial break.

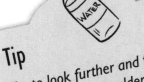

Tip

Try to look further and further over your shoulder each time you look left or right. But do it gently!

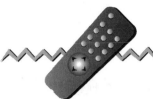

Stretch 2: Neck and Spine

1. Sit backward on a chair or sit cross-legged on the floor.

2. Place your hands, palms down, behind your buttocks with elbows straight but not locked. Your fingertips should hang over the edge of the chair or should be flat on the floor pointing away from you.

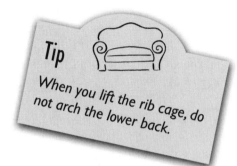

Tip

When you lift the rib cage, do not arch the lower back.

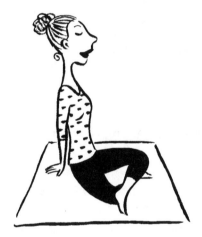

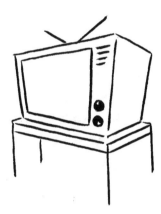

3. Press down through the heels of your hands and inhale as you try to sit taller. Lift your chin and chest toward the ceiling. Do not lock your elbows. Keep them slightly bent.

4. Exhale as you return to a neutral sitting position.

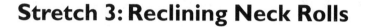

Stretch 3: Reclining Neck Rolls

1. Lie on your back on the floor with your arms at your sides and with your legs either stretched out or with the knees bent, feet flat on the floor.

2. Look at the ceiling. Inhale.

3. Exhale as you allow your head to roll gently to the right.

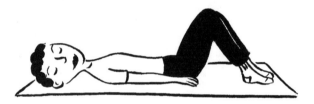

4. Bring your head slowly back to center and repeat this stretch to the left.

5. Continue, alternating right and left, for one commercial.

Challenging Option. Once your neck muscles are relaxed, lift your head by tucking your chin to your chest. Hold this position for a count of three. Relax. Repeat the exercise through one commercial.

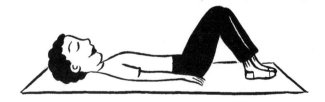

Mid-Back and Under
the Shoulder Blades

The mid-back and shoulder blade area is another favorite stress refuge. After a day of driving, playing computer solitaire (oops! we meant to say, "working at your desk"), and sitting through interminable meetings, the mid-back and shoulder blade area can get really cranky. We feel your pain! Try these exercises for some relief.

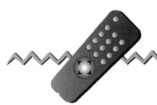

Stretch 4: Upper Back and Shoulders

1. While sitting or standing, stretch your arms straight out in front of you, parallel to the floor. Inhale.

2. Clasp your hands together. Keeping them clasped, turn your hands inside out so that your palms are pointing away from your chest. Round your upper back.

3. Rest your chin on your chest and exhale through the stretch.

4. Keeping your hands flexed, stretch your arms in front of you, as if someone were pulling your palms away from your chest. Feel the stretch through your upper back and shoulders. Exhale as you hold the position.

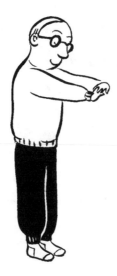

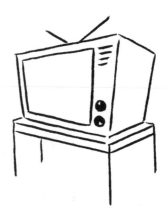

5. Hold the stretch through one commercial and maintain a comfortable breathing pattern. To feel a better stretch, pull the belly button toward your spine and curve your back.

Stretch 5: Upper Back and Shoulders with a Twist

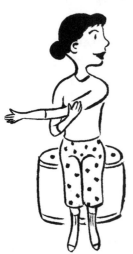

1. While sitting or standing with proper posture, look over your right shoulder. Inhale.

2. Exhale as you use your left hand to pull your right arm across your chest as you try to look behind your right shoulder. Hold for one commercial. Continue breathing regularly.

3. Repeat with the other arm for the next commercial.

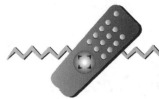

Stretch 6: Upper Back Slide

1. Get on your hands and knees on the floor. Keep your abdominal muscles firm and your head in alignment with your spine.

2. Turn your left hand so that your palm is up.

3. Slide your left arm under your body and between your right arm and right leg.

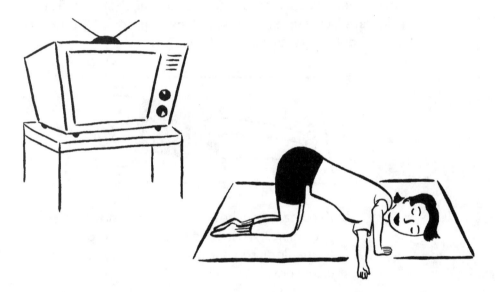

4. Keep your left arm on the floor. Feel the stretch in the upper back.

5. Hold this position for one commercial. Repeat on the other side for the next commercial.

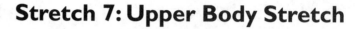

Stretch 7: Upper Body Stretch

While you are on the floor, you may as well try another relaxing stretch for the shoulder area. The shoulders are frequent depositories of stress, so it makes sense to learn as many ways as possible to relieve the tension.

1. Lie flat on your back. Your legs should be flat on the floor.

2. Place your arms so your elbows are bent at right angles and your upper arms are perpendicular to your shoulders. The palms are facing up. (Think, "stick 'em up, pardner!") Your forearms should be resting on the floor.

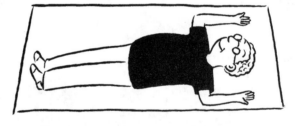

Tip

Draw your shoulder blades down and back. Don't shrug your shoulders!

3. Keeping your elbows on the floor, slowly raise your hands, wrists, and forearms and rotate them to the floor so your hands end up by your hips, palms down.

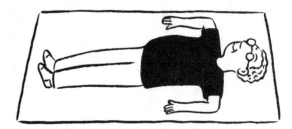

4. Repeat this slowly through one or two commercials.

Lower Back

Lower back pain is the most common complaint among American adults ages 35 to 55. Our evolution from quadrupeds to bipeds was great for human progress, if only because it served as a boon to manufacturers of heating pads, cold packs, and pain relievers. Here are a few stretches to help relieve some of the stress attributed to lower back pain.

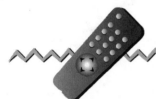

Stretch 8: Lower- and Mid-Back "Cat" Stretch

1. Get on the floor on your hands and knees.

2. Inhale as you arch your back. Allow your head and neck to relax completely and hang toward the floor. Your chin should be on your chest.

DO THIS:

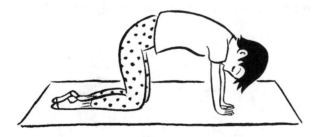

3. Exhale as you reverse this position. Slowly stretch your chest toward the floor and lift your head so there is a slight arch in your back. Your abdominal muscles create the arch. Keep your head neutral.

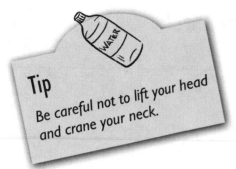

Tip
Be careful not to lift your head and crane your neck.

NOT THIS:

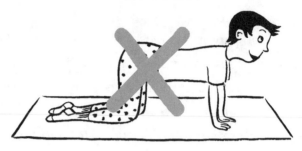

Head lifted too high, too little of an arch

4. Repeat this movement through one commercial.

Stretch 9: Leg Pull

1. Lie on your back with your knees bent and your feet flat on the floor.

2. Place your hands under your knees on the back of your thighs. Inhale.

3. Exhale as you pull your knees to your chest. Your back should be flat on the floor, from your head to your shoulders to your tailbone.

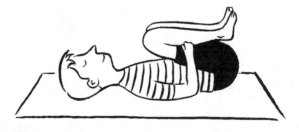

4. Hold the stretch for one commercial and continue breathing gently.

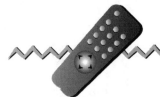

Stretch 10: Back Curve

1. Kneel on the floor so your butt is resting on your heels.

2. Bend at the waist and reach your arms in front of you as you allow your upper body to sink slowly down toward your thighs.

3. Breathe deeply as you sink closer and closer to the floor. As you exhale, relax your muscles and feel the stretch.

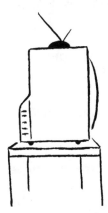

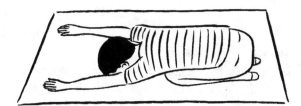

4. After one commercial, circle your arms (keeping them on the floor) so they are next to your legs, palms up. Continue to breathe deeply. Hold for another commercial.

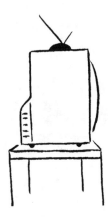

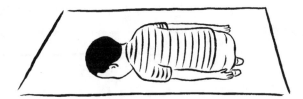

Hips, Butt, and Legs

Because humans do a lot of sitting, the muscles of the hip, butt, and leg often become misaligned. The following stretches are designed to improve the alignment of those muscle groups.

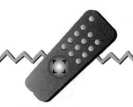

Stretch 11: Hips and Butt

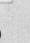

Tip

Be sure to keep your upper back, shoulders, and hips on the floor as much as possible. In other words, don't roll toward the stretch. Instead, turn your head so you are looking away from the stretch.

1. Lie on the floor on your back with your knees bent and your feet flat on the floor.

2. Keeping your right knee bent, straighten your left leg so it lays on the floor.

3. Place your right ankle by the inside of your left thigh. Inhale.

4. Exhale as you relax your right knee over your left leg toward the floor. Keep your shoulder blades on the floor.

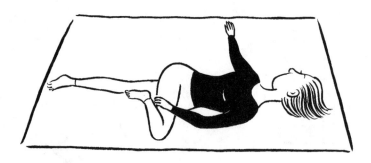

5. Place your left hand on your right knee and apply a gentle pressure. Exhale.

6. Repeat on the other side.

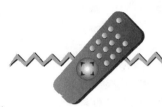

Stretch 12: Hamstrings

Hamstrings are those muscles between your hip joint and knee joint along the back of the leg.

1. Lie on your back with one knee bent, foot flat on the floor. The other leg should be stretched out straight away from your body.

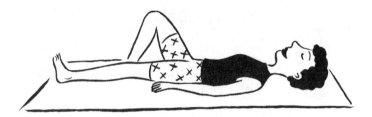

2. Inhale as you lift the straight leg up in the air. Be sure to use those strong abdominal muscles to lift your leg!

3. Place your hands behind the thigh of your lifted leg. Exhale as you gently pull the leg toward your chest (keep the foot flexed to stretch the calf muscles).

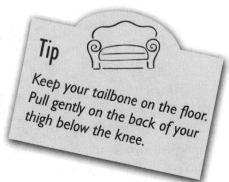

Tip

Keep your tailbone on the floor. Pull gently on the back of your thigh below the knee.

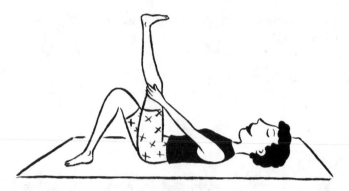

Optional Stretch. Stretch and flex your feet, ankles, and calves by alternately pointing your toes, and then your heels, toward the ceiling. Making circles with your feet while in this position will help with ankle flexibility.

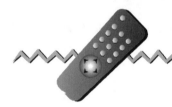

Stretch 13: Quadriceps

1. Lie on your stomach with your hands and arms by your sides. Rest your forehead on the floor.

2. Bend your right leg. Reach back with your right arm and grab the top of your foot. Inhale as you gently pull the heel toward your butt.

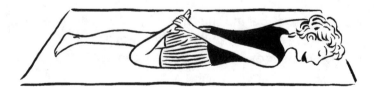

3. Hold the stretch for 15–20 seconds (about one commercial), breathing gently. Keep your hips on the floor.

4. Exhale as you lower your leg. Inhale as you switch to the other leg. Repeat.

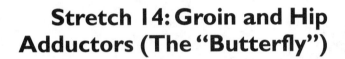

Stretch 14: Groin and Hip Adductors (The "Butterfly")

1. Sit on the floor with the soles of your feet together, spine and head in proper alignment.

2. Hold your ankles with your hands and slowly press your knees toward the floor.

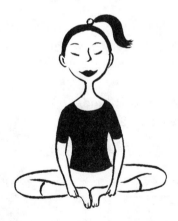

Optional Stretch: If you don't feel this stretch through the groin and hip area, try leaning forward, keeping your spine and head in alignment.

Chest and Arms

We humans operate in the sagital plane for most of our waking life: driving, writing, typing, cooking, and so forth. Too often this wreaks havoc with our posture and, as a consequence, makes the muscles in the chest become too short in relation to the opposing muscles of the upper and mid-back. This stretch helps both as an aid to better posture and as a great stretch for tight chest muscles.

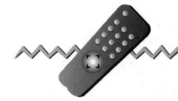

Stretch 15: Chest

1. Stand in a doorway with one of your forearms and palm of the hand against the doorjamb. Your arm will form a 90-degree angle to your body. Inhale.

2. Walk forward gently until you feel the muscles in your chest stretch. Keep your shoulders down and relaxed. Do not shrug them up to your ears.

3. Exhale while counting to 10, and then switch to the other arm.

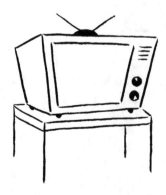

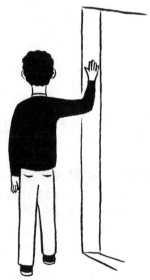

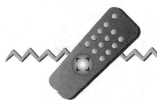

Stretch 16: Triceps

Because we walk with our arms at our sides, the triceps muscles (located at the back of the arms) are in a slightly flexed state most of the day. This stretch will give them a little relief.

1. Place your hand behind your head and reach down between the middle of your shoulder blades (as if there were an "itch" in the middle of your back that you were trying to scratch). Your elbow will be pointing toward the ceiling.

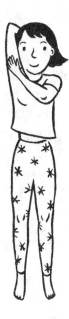
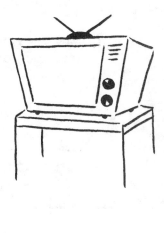

2. Place your other hand so it is pressing gently against the triceps of the opposite arm.

3. Take a deep breath. Exhale slowly. You will feel a stretch along the back of your arm.

Mid-Trunk

These exercises are especially beneficial after doing crunches (chapter 6). They also feel good in the chest and lower back.

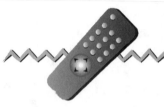

Stretch 17: Abdominal

1. Lie on your stomach. Place your hands beneath you by your shoulders. Inhale.

2. Exhale as you lift your chest gently off the floor. Keep your forearms and elbows on the floor.

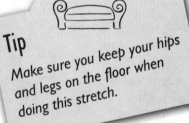

Tip
Make sure you keep your hips and legs on the floor when doing this stretch.

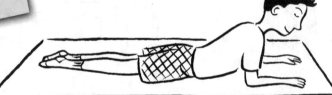

3. Keep your head neutral, not thrown back or tilted forward. Lift through your ribcage.

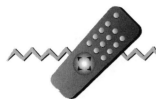

Stretch 18: Waist Twist

Let's face it—sitting in a chair is tedious. A good way to relieve mid-trunk stress and fatigue is with this stretch.

1. Sit in a firm chair (so that you do not "sink"). Fold your arms in front of you. Keep your shoulders relaxed.

2. Inhale while twisting your torso to the right. Follow the twist with your eyes until you are not able to twist any further. Keep your hips pointing forward (do not twist them with the torso).

3. Exhale as you hold the twist. Keep your butt firmly planted on the chair. Continue to breathe through the stretch. With each exhale, relax your back just a little bit more.

4. Hold your position for one commercial or for a count of ten. Repeat to the left side.

chapter four

Gettin' Pushy

How to Firm Your Chest, Back, Shoulders, and Arms

Now that you've checked your posture, assessed your balance, learned how to breathe, and stretched, you are ready to begin the muscle-fitness portion of the book.

As we discussed in chapter 1, acquiring more muscle (more lean tissue) can mean the difference between aging gracefully and aging abruptly. After the age of twenty, an inactive person loses about *half a pound* of muscle per year. We do not advocate this type of weight loss! Here's why.

One pound of muscles requires 50 calories to maintain itself; one pound of fat only requires 3 calories. This is why a person with more fat tissue has more difficulty losing weight regardless of the number of calories being consumed (or not consumed) than the person with more muscle. According to Covert Bailey, author of *Smart Exercise*, muscle is a veritable "calorie furnace." The more muscle you have, the more fuel (calories) your body requires to maintain itself.

Many women worry that strength exercises will turn them into knuckle-dragging hulks. Not so. You will not wake up one day looking like someone dressed you in George Clooney's "Bat Suit." You will, however, start to feel stronger and firmer. As for you guys out there, give yourself a break and start back to studville slowly by doing wall, kitchen counter, and knee pushups for a few weeks before jumping right to the classic hands and toes pushup position. Your back and shoulder joints will thank you for your restraint!

We have choreographed ten easy-to-follow strengthening exercises for the upper body. Each individual exercise can be done during one commercial break. Your goal is to do each specific ex-

Remember!

There is no such thing as "spot-reducing." Working on a specific area of the body, such as the thighs or abdominals, will not necessarily result in fat loss from that area. Expending more energy while consuming fewer calories, however, will result in the loss of body fat throughout the body. This may or may not mean that the fat will disappear immediately from the area you are targeting, but if you are consistent with proper diet and exercise, eventually your body will grant you your wish!

ercise for an entire commercial break. The exercises are shown in order, from the easiest to the more difficult, so be sure to go at a pace that is comfortable for you. When performing pushups, keep your head neutral. It should not be looking up, nor should your chin be tucked into your chest. Instead your spine and neck should remain in alignment. If you need to, refer to chapter 2 for a refresher on good posture versus bad posture.

Chest

Doing pushups is the most effective way to strengthen and condition the upper body without spending a fortune on exercise equipment. Pushups primarily benefit the chest, shoulders, and arms. The abdominal muscles and the back muscles play an assisting and supporting role.

Isometrics

As an alternative to pushups, we suggest that great "Charles Atlas" exercise from fifty years ago: isometrics. Simply place your hands together in front of you in either a "prayer" position (palms together) or knuckles together. Breathe normally as you push the heels of your hands or knuckles together. Squeeze as hard as you can for an entire commercial. Increase the difficulty by adding commercials until you can do this exercise for an entire commercial break. But don't hunch up those shoulders. Keep them down and relaxed.

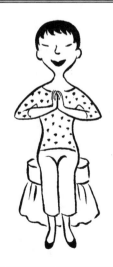

The easiest way to learn to do pushups and feel their benefits is to do the exercise against a wall or kitchen counter. Be sure to check your hands for telltale snack debris first!

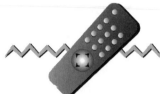

Exercise 1: Wall Pushups

DO THIS:

NOT THIS:

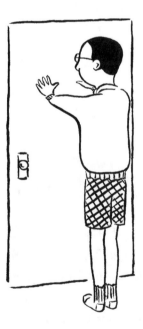

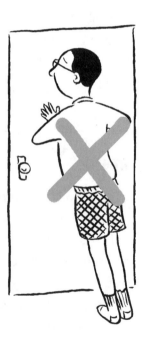

Spine straight, elbows parallel
to the ground, head neutral

Elbows down, back swayed,
head drooping

1. Stand facing the wall with your feet shoulder-width apart (about 6 inches).

2. Extend your arms in front of you at about shoulder height and shoulder-width apart. Your arms should be parallel to the floor.

3. Place your hands on the wall, fingers spread apart and pointing toward the ceiling. Your feet should be 6 to 8 inches more than an arm's length from the wall.

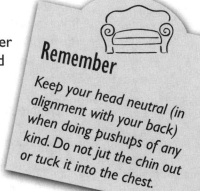

Remember

Keep your head neutral (in alignment with your back) when doing pushups of any kind. Do not jut the chin out or tuck it into the chest.

4. Pull your shoulders back and down and bring your shoulder blades together. Tighten your stomach muscles and press your chest toward the wall. Do not arch your back. Your feet should be either flat on the floor or with heels slightly lifted, whichever is more comfortable.

5. Continue to look straight ahead. Inhale, keep your stomach muscles tight, and bend your arms as you lower your body toward the wall.

6. Be sure to keep your arms parallel to the floor and your elbows in line with your shoulders.

7. Exhale as you push away from the wall.

Suggested Program. The first time you try this exercise, perform as many as you can during the first commercial. Then, each subsequent time you do the exercise, add another commercial until you can do the wall pushups for an entire commercial break (about 2 to 3 minutes ... but who's counting?). Once this becomes easy, you are ready for the more difficult pushups to follow.

Challenging Option. Instead of doing pushups against a wall, use the kitchen counter or another solid piece of furniture, allowing your body to be at an increased angle. This will provide more of a challenge (and you won't have to clean any handprints off the wall).

Troubleshooting

• You may need to experiment with the exact positions of your arms and legs. Use the first commercial break to adjust your form.

• You should feel the muscles working in your chest, upper back, and shoulder areas when you do this exercise.

• If you feel any pain or discomfort in your shoulders, look at your elbow positions. Your elbows and arms should be parallel to the floor. Your elbows should *not* point toward the floor as you bend your arms.

Exercise 2: All-Fours Pushups

This exercise serves as a stepping-stone between Wall Pushups and Knee Pushups (Exercise 3).

DO THIS:

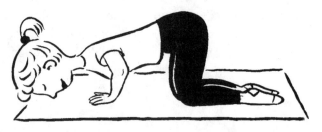

Head neutral, abdominal muscles tight, back straight

NOT THIS:

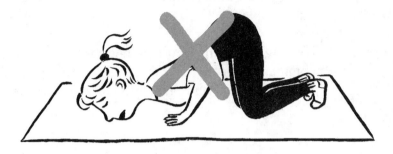

Back swayed, chin jutting out

1. Get on the floor on your hands and knees.

2. Keeping your abdominal muscles tight, your back straight, and your head neutral, inhale as you lower your chest, shoulders, and head toward the floor. Your elbows should point away from your body at a 90° angle.

3. Exhale as you push yourself back to the all-fours position.

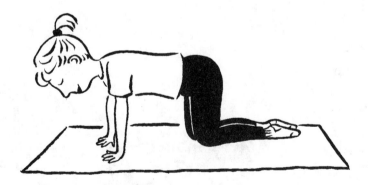

4. Do this exercise for one commercial.

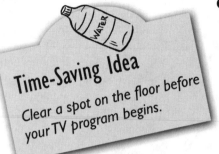

Challenging Option. As you get stronger, try to do the All-Fours Pushups through an entire commercial break.

Troubleshooting. You may need to use the first commercial break to experiment with the positioning of your hands in relation to your shoulders.

Time-Saving Idea
Clear a spot on the floor before your TV program begins.

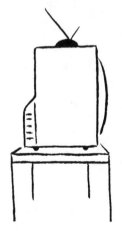

Exercise 3: Knee Pushups

By performing Wall Pushups and All-Fours Pushups, you have built the foundation for a stronger upper body. This next exercise will continue building on that foundation to help you increase your strength.

DO THIS:

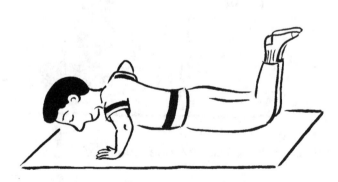

Head neutral, abdominal muscles tight, spine straight

NOT THIS:

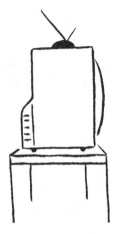

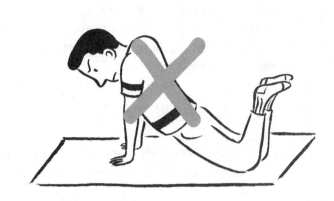

Chin on chest, back swayed

1. Lie on your stomach on the floor.

2. Keeping your thighs on the floor, bend your knees so that your shins are perpendicular to the floor (your feet should be pointing toward the ceiling).

3. Place the palms of your hands 6–8 inches to the outside of your shoulders and flat on the floor. Inhale.

4. Tighten your abdominal muscles and exhale as you push yourself away from the floor.

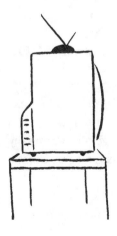

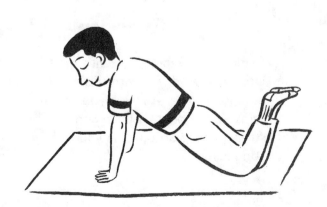

5. Inhale as you lower yourself back to the floor. Repeat as many times as you can during the commercial break.

Challenging Option. Instead of allowing your body to go all the way to the floor, stop just as your chin and chest get within an inch of the floor, then push up again. Do not allow your body to rest on the floor.

Troubleshooting

- When pushups are done correctly, you should feel the muscles in your chest, back, abdomen, arms, and shoulders.

- Your head, neck, and back should be in a straight line . . . no swayed back, no butt sticking up in the air, and no head flopping!

- Keep your abdominal muscles tight. (This will help with the previous item in this list.)

- If you feel any pain in your shoulders, recheck the position of your hands in relation to your shoulders. Your hands should be in line with your shoulders, not with your head or chest.

Exercise 4: Elevated Pushups

Rather than leaping right into the Classic Pushups, why not work into them gradually with this exercise? Elevated pushups are excellent for strengthening your chest, shoulders, upper back, and arms. As a bonus, your abdominal muscles get good secondary strengthening. So, build up your strength with this exercise before continuing.

You'll need a low couch, hassock, footstool, large pillow, cushion, or futon. Start with something that is only about a foot high and is comfortable and soft enough to put your knees on.

DO THIS:

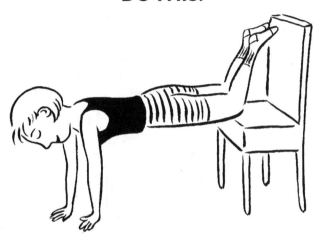

Head neutral, abdominal muscles tight, spine straight, elbows soft

NOT THIS:

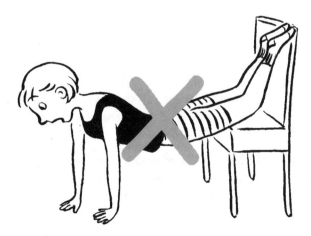

Back swayed, chin jutting, elbows locked

1. Place your knees on the stool or couch and extend your body across the floor. You will be supporting yourself with your hands, which should be shoulder-width apart, with your fingers spread apart and pointing forward.

2. Keeping your abdominal muscles tight and your body properly aligned, inhale as you lower yourself until your chin is near the floor.

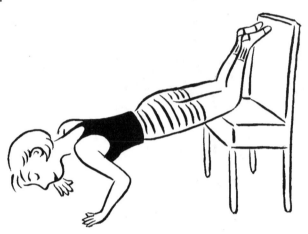

3. Exhale as you push back to the starting position. Your elbows should be straight but not locked, and your shoulders should be relaxed, not shrugged around your ears.

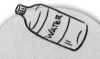

Commercial Break

Every time you see a fast-food commercial, do a set of push-ups. Imagine that you are pushing that fast food away from you as you get healthy and happy.

Suggested Program. Do this exercise for one commercial, rest for the next commercial, and then repeat the exercise for the third commercial.

Ultimate Challenge. Do Elevated Pushups for an entire commercial break.

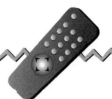

Exercise 5: Classic Pushups

Don't feel discouraged if this particular type of pushup is difficult for you to do. Classic Pushups (also known as military pushups) require a great deal of strength in the chest, back, shoulders, abdominal muscles, and arms. If you feel like your back sways when attempting this exercise, stick with Elevated Pushups instead.

DO THIS:

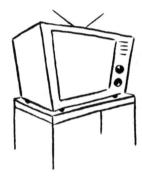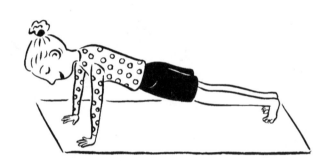

Arms directly under shoulders, body in a
straight line from head to heels

NOT THIS:

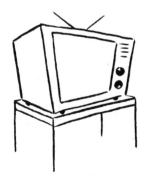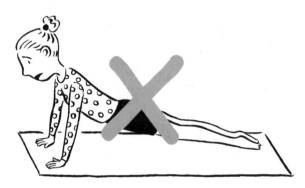

Back swayed, chin jutting toward the floor, feet pointed

1. Extend your legs behind you. Your feet should be close to-gether and flexed, with the weight on the balls of your feet for support.

2. Place your arms shoulder-width apart, fingers spread apart.

3. Keeping your head neutral, chin not tucked or tilted and hips and butt "straight," inhale as you lower yourself to the floor.

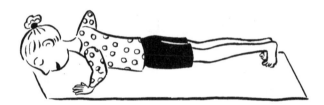

4. Exhale as you push yourself away from the floor until your arms are straight. Again, do not lock your elbows.

Ultimate Challenge. Properly execute Classic Pushups for one or two entire commercials. This is quite an accomplishment! Congratulate your-self!

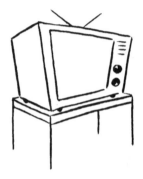

Variation

If you are having trouble push-ing yourself up from the floor, then try this variation: Simply lower yourself down to the floor as slowly as you can. Relax, get back into position, and do it again.

Back

After all of the muscle action with the chest, shoulder, and arm muscles, it's a good idea to pay some specific attention to the back muscles. The best back exercises involve gym equipment, such as pull-down machines, seated rowing machines, and chinning bars. Assuming the absence of a personal home gym (and because pushups do involve the back muscles quite a bit), the following exercises will help stretch, strengthen, and balance your upper torso by gently flexing your back, especially your lower back.

Because you will be face down on the floor for this exercise, your first task is to get out the vacuum cleaner and tidy up a spot for yourself. Take note of "dust bunny" locations for future cleaning adventures. Vacuuming is great exercise, too!

Exercise 6: The "X"

1. Lie face down on the floor. Keep your head neutral. Stretch your arms out in front of you.

2. Keeping your head in alignment with your spine, lift your right arm and left leg. Breathe normally. Hold for one commercial.

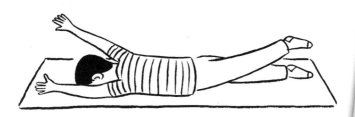

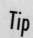
Tip

To keep your head neutral in the back strengthening exercise, rest your forehead on the floor. As you lift your arms and legs, the head should lift but should remain in alignment with the spine.

3. Next lift your left arm and right leg and hold for one commercial. Keep your hips squarely on the floor.

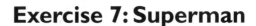

Exercise 7: Superman

1. While lying face down on the floor, stretch both arms out in front of you. Lift both arms at the same time, just like Superman "flying" through the air, and hold for one commercial. Keep your hips and legs on the floor.

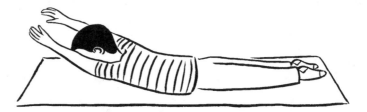

2. Reverse this by putting the arms down and lifting both legs. Hold for one commercial.

3. It is very important that you keep your abdominal and gluteal muscles tight throughout this exercise.

Triceps

The following exercises are particularly effective for the area on the back of the arms, or as Bette Midler once said, "The part that keeps waving long after you have stopped waving good-bye." Tightening and toning the muscles in this area is important for those of us who want to enjoy wearing anything sleeveless.

Exercise 8: Triceps Wall Pushups

The body position for this exercise is similar to Exercise 1, but the change in hand position makes it a completely different exercise.

DO THIS: **NOT THIS:**

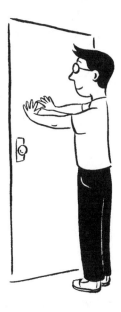

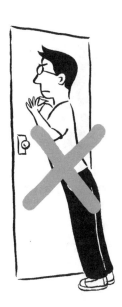

Back and head in alignment, elbows pointing away from shoulders

Back swayed, elbows pointing toward the floor

1. Place your hands side by side on the wall, fingers spread apart. Unlike Exercise 1, move your hands so you form a small triangle with your thumbs and forefingers. Keep those fingers spread apart!

2. Your feet should be about 6–8 inches more than an arm's length from the wall and either flat on the floor or with your heels slightly lifted, whichever is more comfortable.

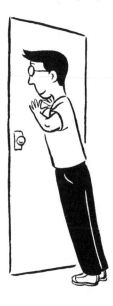

3. Inhale as you lower yourself toward the wall. Your arms and elbows should remain parallel to the floor. Don't drop those elbows.

4. Exhale as you push away from the wall until you have returned to the start position (without locking the elbows).

Suggested Program. Do this exercise for an entire commercial break. You will be amazed at how tight your arms feel!

Troubleshooting

Commercial Break

When you see a commercial for a housecleaning product, do a set of triceps exercises. For the next housecleaning commercial, do a set of biceps exercises. This will get you in shape for your own housecleaning work!

• If you feel any pain in your neck and shoulders, make sure you haven't inadvertently hunched your shoulders around your neck.

• It is important to straighten your arms to get full benefit from this exercise. Be sure to push yourself away from the wall in a controlled fashion—gently—without locking your elbows.

The "dip," a common exercise for the triceps, is omitted from our book because it can be very rough on the shoulder joints and wrists. Instead, you will find the next three exercises equally as challenging and just as effective.

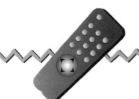

Exercise 9: Single-Arm
Triceps Pushups

1. Lie on your right side, with your right elbow bent and the right hand and forearm resting on your stomach. Your left hand should be palm down on the floor in front of your midsection. Legs are together, knees bent slightly. Inhale.

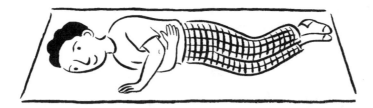

2. Exhale as you press down with your left hand until your shoulder lifts off the floor and your right arm swings freely. Keep your head in alignment with your spine. Do not turn your head to the left or right.

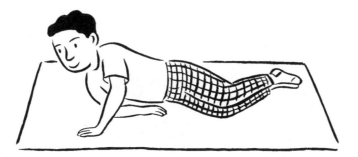

3. Keep pressing until your left arm straightens. Do not lock your elbow.

4. Lower yourself back to the floor as you inhale.

Suggested Program. Do each arm for one product commercial. When that becomes easy, repeat through several commercials for each side.

Troubleshooting

- *Never* allow your elbows to "snap" into place when you push yourself away from the floor.

- Always push from the *heel of the hand,* not from the palm.

- Posture is very important. Keep your head in a neutral position. Look straight ahead and keep your back straight.

Exercise 10: Elevated Triceps Pushups

DO THIS:

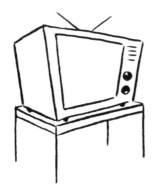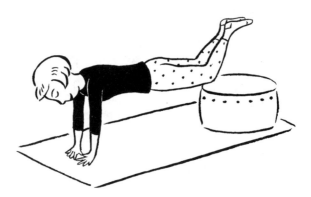

Back and head in alignment; elbows pointed away from body,
not toward feet; abdominal muscles tight

NOT THIS:

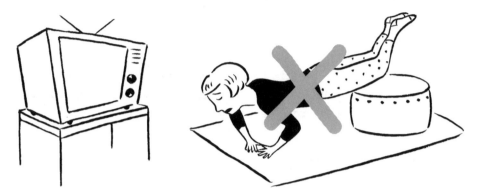

Back bowed, chin jutting toward the floor, knees too far back on chair

This exercise is similar to Elevated Pushups (Exercise 4), except for the position of the hands.

1. With your knees on a couch or hassock, place your hands on the floor under your shoulders. Your thumbs and fore-fingers should be touching and forming a small triangle (as in Exercise 8).

2. Slowly lower yourself to the floor by bending your elbows, pointing them away from you. Inhale.

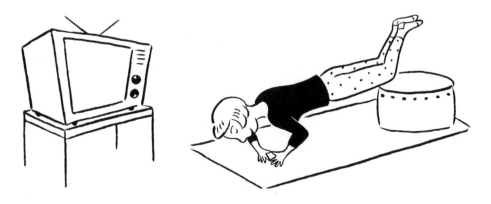

3. Your back should be straight. Keep your abdominal muscles tight and your head neutral.

4. Exhale as you push back to the starting position.

Suggested Program. Do this exercise through as many commercials as possible. Your ultimate goal is to do this exercise through an entire commercial break.

Troubleshooting

- *Never* allow your elbows to "snap" into place when you push yourself away from the floor.

- Always push through the *heel of the hand,* not from the palm or the fingers.

- Posture is very important. Keep your head in a neutral position. Look directly at the floor and keep your back straight.

Exercise 11: Classic Triceps Pushups

DO THIS:

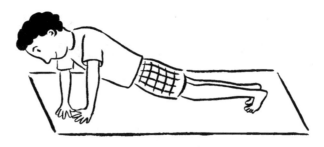

Straight line from head to heels, elbows pointing
directly away from shoulders

NOT THIS:

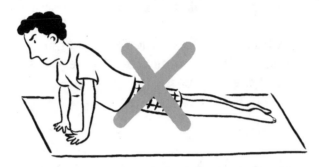

Back swayed, shoulders hunched up around neck,
chin lifted too high, feet pointeed

1. Lie on your stomach and extend your legs behind you. Flex your feet and put your weight on the balls of your feet.

2. Your arms should be under your chest with your fingers spread. Your thumbs and first fingers form a triangle.

3. Keeping your head neutral, chin not tucked or tilted, and your hips and butt "straight," inhale as you lower yourself to the floor.

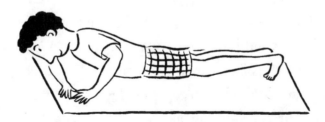

4. Exhale as you push yourself away from the floor until your arms are straight. Again, do not lock your elbows.

Suggested Program. Do this exercise for one commercial, rest for one commercial, and do it again for one commercial.

Ultimate Challenge. Do Classic Triceps Pushups for an entire commercial break. This is no mean feat! Give yourself a high five and a couple of chest thumps!

Troubleshooting

- Use your whole hand for the pushup and push through the heel of the hand. Keep your hands flat on the floor throughout the entire range of motion.

- Keep your back, neck, and head in proper alignment—no swayed backs or arched necks!

- Do not "snap" your elbows into a locked position. Straighten your arms gently as you push away from the floor.

Biceps

The biceps are the two muscles at the front of the arm between the shoulder and the elbow. While images of World Wrestling Federation stars flexing massive arms are what usually spring to mind when we think of biceps, the fact is that we cannot even pick up our car keys (let alone pick up "The Rock") without using our biceps. Strengthening this muscle group without the use of equipment means a visit, once again, with that old master of yore, Charles Atlas. He discovered that by pitting one muscle against another (which he called "dynamic tension"), he could increase the muscle's strength and size. The following exercise can be done while seated or standing.

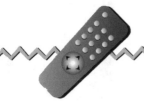

Exercise 12: Isometric Biceps Curls

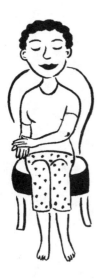

1. Reach your left arm across your body and place the heel of your left hand on the heel of your right hand.

2. Try to bend your right arm up toward your shoulder while pressing down with the left arm.

3. As you lower the arm, use the right hand to create resistance against the left hand. This way you get a good workout coming and going.

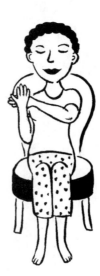

Suggested Program. Do this for one commercial and repeat on the other arm for the next commercial. Keep switching from left arm to right arm for the entire commercial break.

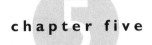

chapter five

Spin Your Wheels!

Great Exercises for Your Legs

Because the leg muscles are the largest muscle group in the body, we have divided the exercises in this chapter into three categories: the quadriceps (front of the leg between the hip and the knee); the hamstrings (back of the leg between the butt and the knee); and the calves (back of the leg between the knee and the heel).

Strong, stable leg muscles are the essence of mobility. Practically speaking, getting up from a chair, sitting down on the toilet, and walking up and down stairs are everyday tasks that require strong leg muscles. But it's not just a matter of function, is it? We all want the legs of Tina Turner or Magnum, P.I.! Let's face it, when summer rolls around, we want our legs to look their best in those swimsuits and shorts!

The following exercises are designed for pragmatism as well as pulchritude (a heavy-duty word that means "seriously foxy"). Each of the exercises in the specific categories progresses from easier to more difficult. Go at your own pace, and concentrate on good form. Don't go through all of the exercises at once. Be patient with yourself and move on to more difficult exercises *only* if your comfort level permits!

Let's get going!

Quadriceps

Even though these exercises mainly target the muscles at the front of your thighs, keep in mind that the hamstrings, gluteal muscles (of the buttocks), and calves will also come into play.

Exercise 1: Chair Squats

Getting up out of a chair should be a nonthreatening activity. For several million Americans, however, it is an exhausting and daunting task. Chair Squats utilize the leg muscles that are involved in our most basic tasks, such as getting up out of a chair or sitting down on the toilet.

The objective in this exercise is to stand up and sit down without using your arms to assist you. At first, you may feel more secure using your arms. If so, continue to use them until you feel confident enough in the strength of your legs to sit and stand unassisted. You will feel the quadriceps muscles primarily with this exercise.

DO THIS:

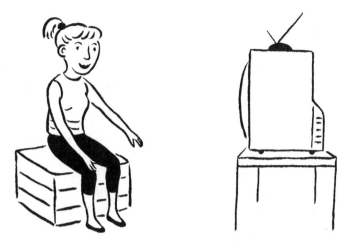

Head neutral, shoulders back, chest open, curve in lower back so
the butt is sliding back toward the chair, knees over ankles

NOT THIS:

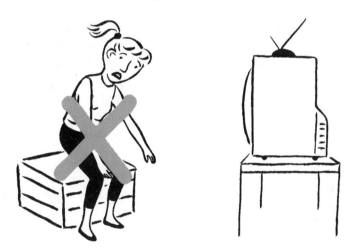

Head looking at floor, shoulders rounded, waist bent so
that torso is at 45 degrees, knees bent over toes

1. Start in a sitting position. Keep your abdominal muscles tight and your head neutral as you lift your chest. Make sure you don't arch your back.

2. With feet shoulder-width apart, lean forward slightly, and push through your heels to a standing position. Exhale as you stand.

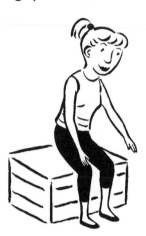 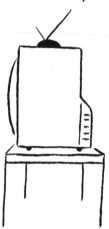

3. Using the muscles in your legs to control your descent, sit sloooowwwwwly back into your seat. Inhale as you sit down. As you sit back, do not point the knees over your toes. Instead, your knees should remain above your heels and your shins should be perpendicular to the floor. This will make your butt stick out behind you as you sit down into the chair.

Suggested Program. Repeat this exercise for an entire commercial break.

Tip

When squatting, do NOT bend the knees first. Instead concentrate on lowering your hips and butt back behind the heels of the feet. This will cause your knees to bend naturally.

Troubleshooting

- If you feel any discomfort in your knees, check your head and your knee positions. Looking down at your feet can place too much of your body weight on the balls of your feet, which may cause knee discomfort. The knees should not travel over the toes; concentrate on keeping your shins perpendicular to the floor.

- Be sure that you are always looking straight ahead and are keeping your weight mainly on your heels, especially when standing up.

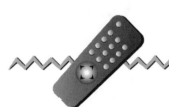

Exercise 2: Pulsing Lunges

Lunges are great exercises for the quadriceps, hamstring, and gluteal (butt) muscles (for more butt exercises, see chapter 6). For lunges, you may need to hold on to the back of a sturdy chair or sofa until you feel secure doing this exercise without support. The term "lunge" often creates a mental picture of Zorro thrusting forward with a sword while fighting the Evil Villain. For this exercise, however, think "plunge" (up and down like a bathroom plunger, only slower). In other words, you will be moving vertically, not horizontally. This image should help you keep your knees and back safe.

DO THIS:

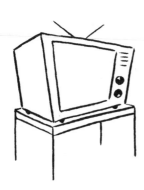
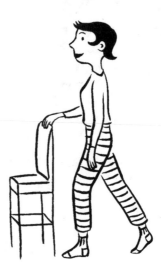

Head neutral, chest open, shoulders back, forward knee over ankle, back leg
supported by ball of foot, back heel aligned with back knee

NOT THIS:

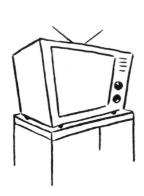
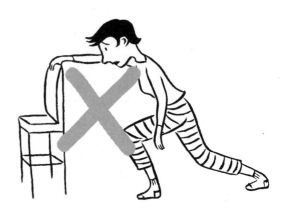

Head down, shoulders rounded, knee ahead of toes on front leg,
foot skewed sideways with heel of back leg pointing inward

1. Stand beside your sturdy chair, one hand holding firmly onto the chair. Your left leg should be beneath you, and your right leg should be back behind you. Your feet should be about a stride-width apart.

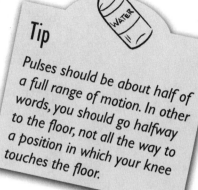

Tip

Pulses should be about half of a full range of motion. In other words, you should go halfway to the floor, not all the way to a position in which your knee touches the floor.

2. Your left foot should be flat on the floor. The weight of your right foot should be on the ball of that foot with toes in line with your knee, not pointing away or to the side.

3. Inhale as you bend your left leg so the knee of your right leg bends toward the floor a few inches. Your left knee should not go forward over your toes! Keep your left shin perpendicular to the ground.

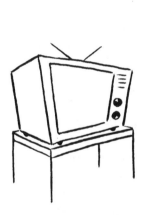 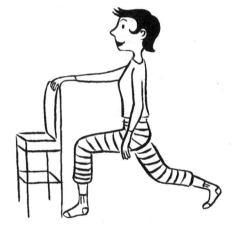

4. Exhale as you slowly push yourself back to a standing position. Push from your left leg's heel and balance from the ball of your right leg. Keep your knees slightly bent throughout the exercise—do not lock them.

5. Repeat, or pulse, ten times.

6. Do another ten pulses by stepping backward with your right leg.

DRINK WATER!

Suggested Program. Do as many repetitions as possible through a commercial break. Keep your pace steady, slow, and deliberate.

Ultimate Goal. Do pulsing lunges through an entire commercial break. This exercise can be challenging!

Troubleshooting

- When lunging, your knees should never push forward over your toes. Keep your shins as perpendicular to the floor as possible.

- If you are having trouble keeping your balance, hold onto the chair and focus on keeping your weight evenly distributed between both legs. Also, keeping the abdominal muscles tight will help keep you standing straight.

- You should *always* be able to see the toes of the forward leg. If not, then that means your knee is going over your toes!

- Keep looking straight ahead (at the TV commercials, of course). Your posture must be properly aligned (no slouching). There will be a slight curve in your lower back. Imagine that you are lifting your ribcage off of your hipbones.

- Pulse slowly. You aren't churning butter, pumping water, or drilling for oil—take your time. Feel the muscles in your legs working.

- Be mindful of any stress on the knee joints, hips, or ankles.

- Don't forget to breathe! Inhale as your knees bend and exhale as you stand up.

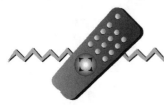

Exercise 3: Step-Ups

For this exercise, you should have a stair step close by or use a very sturdy stool or box no more than 6–8 inches high. Your posture is important, as always. Remember to keep your head neutral and avoid the temptation to look down at your feet. The quadriceps and butt muscles are the primary areas worked in this exercise.

1. Place your *entire* right foot on the step and exhale as you push yourself up, primarily from your right heel. By pushing from the heel of your right foot instead of from the ball of that foot, you will protect your knees from unnecessary stress.

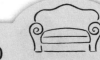

Tip

For all leg exercises, make sure your chest remains open (do not collapse your ribcage) and your shoulder blades come closer together around the spine. Do not shrug your shoulders. Keep your abdominal, lower back, and butt muscles activated.

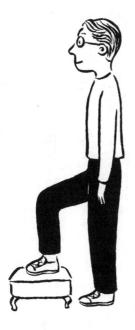 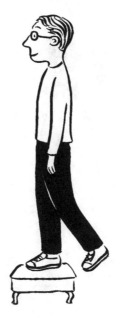

2. Inhale as you return your right foot to the floor. Repeat.

3. Keep doing this exercise with your right leg for one commercial. Switch to your left leg for the next commercial.

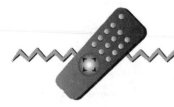

Exercise 4: Sumo Squats

This is a great exercise for the adductors (the muscles of the inner thighs).

DO THIS:

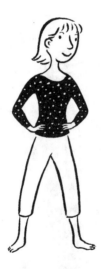
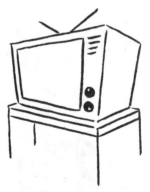

Head neutral, legs wider than shoulders, knees over ankles, slight curve in lower back, butt behind heels, chest open, shoulders back

NOT THIS:

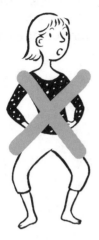 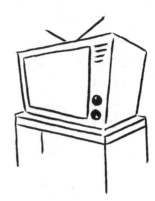

Head down, torso bent forward, knees pushed over toes,
heels lifting off the floor

1. Stand with your legs slightly wider than shoulder-width. Keep your back straight and your knees and toes turned slightly out.

2. Lower yourself straight down toward your heels by pushing your butt down about 45 degrees and no further than 90 degrees. Inhale as you lower your body.

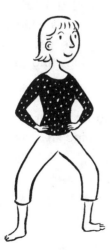 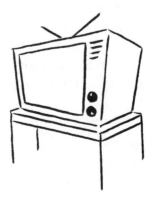

Tip

The position of the knees is of utmost importance when squatting and lunging. Never push your knees beyond the toes of the bent leg. Keep your shins as perpendicular to the floor as possible.

3. With most of the effort coming from your gluteal muscles (as a result of pressing through your heels), return to a standing position as you exhale. Repeat through an entire commercial break.

Exercise 5: Progressive Reverse Lunges with a Slide Pulse

This exercise is similar to Exercise 2, except that instead of remaining in a stationary position with one leg behind the other throughout the move, you will be stepping back a little bit more each time. This will require you to use those balancing skills you learned in chapter 2!

Hold on to a chair or sofa for balance and stability until you feel confident, strong, and stable enough to do this while standing free. Also, continuous stepping and pulsing can get your heart muscle pumping, so be aware of your breathing and be sure to keep hydrated.

1. Start in a standing position. Step back about 12 inches with your right leg (as if you were stepping behind an imaginary line).

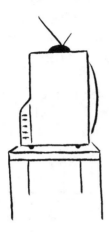
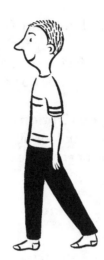

2. Inhale as you lower yourself toward the floor into a lunge position. Pulse two times.

3. Exhale as you push back to the starting position.

4. Now step back in a little bit bigger of a lunge with the same foot. Pulse two times.

5. Finally, step back far enough so you are doing a full lunge position. Pulse two more times.

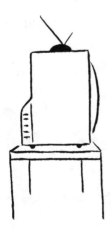
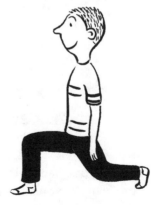

Suggested Program. Do this for one or two commercials, then switch to the left leg for the next couple of commercials. Repeat throughout the entire commercial break, switching legs each time you complete three complete reverse lunges per leg.

Challenging Option. Complete four exercises on each leg. Start with your foot about 12 inches behind you and then build up to a full lunge with each successive exercise.

Hamstrings

This exercise targets the hamstrings (the muscles at the back of the thigh). You will also feel a little action in the butt muscles. The hamstrings are too often ignored or underutilized in many exercise programs. Few people realize how important this muscle group is for maintaining strong, stable knees. The quadriceps are *four* muscles (Remember your Latin? *Quad* = "four"). The hamstrings are only three muscles. If you ignore the hamstrings and work only the quads, your leg muscles risk being out of balance. This means that there could be added pressure placed on the front of your knee, which could result in muscle imbalance or unnecessary strain or injury. So don't ignore your hamstrings!

Exercise 6: Hamstring Pulses

1. Lie on your back with your feet flat on the floor, knees bent, and arms at your sides.

2. Inhale while you straighten your right leg and flex your heel toward the ceiling. Keep your abdominal muscles tight and your head and back flat on the floor.

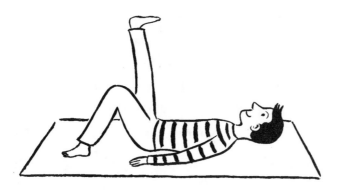

3. Exhale as you lift your hips by pushing down on your left foot through the heel. Imagine you are trying to touch your right foot to the ceiling. Pulse by lifting and lowering your hips and pushing down on your left heel. Breathe regularly. When you lift your hip, make sure your upper back remains on the floor. This will help you avoid putting too much pressure on your neck.

Commercial Break

During the next car commercial, do a set of leg exercises. This way you can build up those leg exercises, enabling you to walk to the store instead of driving!

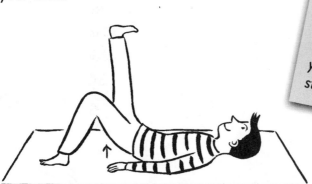

Suggested Program. Continue with the same leg for the entire commercial. Switch legs and repeat for the next commercial.

Calves and Shins

The calf muscles are used extensively when walking, so it makes good sense to keep them strong. Another reward for properly exercising your calves is improved shapeliness, a real plus when wearing shorts next summer! Before we begin working on the calf muscles, however, we want to be sure that the muscles along the shinbone aren't neglected, which is why we start with Toe Taps. Sitting and tapping your toes is exercise . . . who knew?

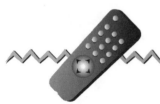

Exercise 7: Toe Taps

Tip

Toe taps are a great exercise to do during the theme song of your favorite show. Just tap those toes in time with the music!

1. While watching your show, lift and lower the balls of your feet, keeping your heels on the floor.

2. "Tap" your toes for a minute or two, and then rest.

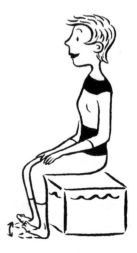

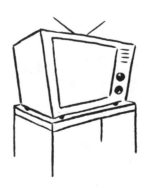

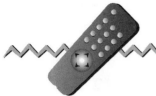

Exercise 8: Basic Calf Raises

This simple exercise can be done standing next to your easy chair.

1. Stand beside a chair. If necessary, hold on to the back of the chair for balance.

2. Exhale as you raise your heels off the floor. Your weight is now on the balls of your feet (tiptoe). Keep your back straight and don't lean back away from the chair. Hold for 2 or 3 seconds.

3. Inhale as you return to the start position.

Suggested Program. At first, repeat the calf raises for only two to three commercials. Add commercials as you feel your calves strengthen.

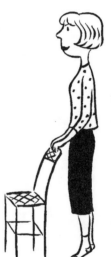

Remember!

Stretch your calves before sitting down! Hold on to the back of a chair. Keep your feet flat on the floor and lean forward slightly. Hold for at least 15 seconds. As another option, you can slightly bend one leg and then the other while pressing back into the heel of your straight leg. You should feel this stretch throughout the length of your calves.

Exercise 9: One-Legged Calf Raises

Proceed to this exercise only when you feel that your calf muscles are strong enough.

1. Stand behind your chair with your left foot on the floor. Bend your right leg so your right foot is completely off the floor.

2. While holding on to the back of the chair, inhale as you raise the heel of your left foot.

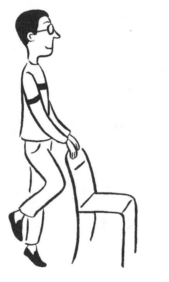 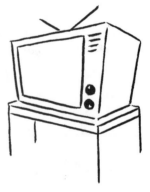

3. Take your time—hold your heel in the raised position for 2 seconds.

4. Exhale as you lower your heel back to the floor.

5. After 15 to 20 repetitions (one to two commercials), switch feet.

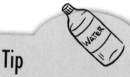

Exercise 10: Calf Raises with Changing Toe Positions

1. Stand on a stair step on the balls of your feet, heels hanging off of the edge (think Greg Louganis at the Olympics as he prepares to do a back flip).

2. If necessary, hold on to a banister for balance. Do calf raises for one commercial.

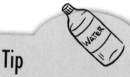

Tip

As a challenging option, do not hold onto anything for support, as shown in the illustrations.

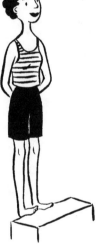

3. For the second commercial, turn your toes out (like Charlie Chaplin) and then do your calf raises.

4. For the third commercial, turn your toes in (like a pigeon) and do your calf raises.

5. Remember to breathe!

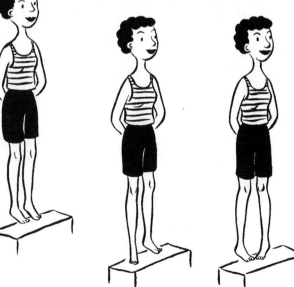

6

Butts
and
Guts

Although "rock-hard" buns and "six-pack" stomachs make great ad copy, few of us can, or should, make this our primary objective when exercising these muscle groups. The butt muscles (gluteus maximus, medius, and minimus) allow us to stand up, walk, and climb stairs. The abdominal muscles are involved in almost every activity we perform. Together, these two muscle groups provide a strong structural unit that assists in maintaining a strong back and good posture. The butt exercises also involve the hamstrings; they are often used in concert with one another.

The following exercises are simple, effective, and easy to do. They will strengthen and shape your muscles. They will not

"spot-reduce" these areas. Be wary of any program that prom-
ises to do that.

The exercises in each category gradually become more difficult, so take your time and go at your own pace.

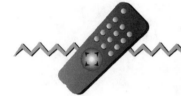

Butt

Exercise 1: Butt Lift-Backs

DO THIS:

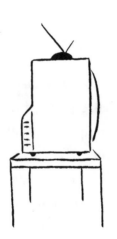 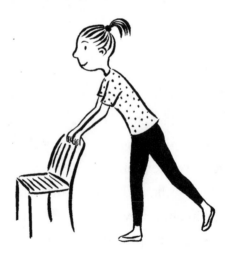

Head neutral, shoulders "square," legs straight,
feet flexed, spine neutral

NOT THIS:

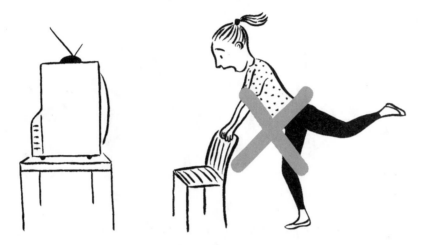

Chin on chest, back overarched, knees bent, toes pointed

1. Stand behind a sturdy chair with your feet hip-width apart.

2. Check your posture. You should be looking straight ahead (at a TV commercial, of course). Use the chair and TV as a "landmark" for your correct body position. No slouching or rocking your body back and forth!

3. Inhale as you lift your leg back behind you. Squeeze your butt muscles to lift your leg. Do not swing your leg in an un-controlled fashion. Your torso should not move.

4. Keep your lifted leg straight (but not locked straight) and your foot flexed. The toes of your standing leg should be pointing toward the chair. The toes of the lifted leg should be pointing toward the floor.

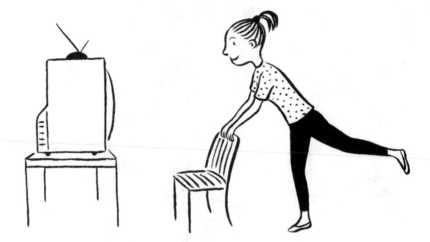

5. Continue to squeeze your butt muscles at the highest point of your lift, holding it there for a count of 3.

6. Exhale as you return to the start position. Repeat with your other leg.

Suggested Program. Continue to alternate legs through an entire commercial break.

Troubleshooting

- It is important to feel the butt muscles, not the back muscles, during the execution of this exercise.

- Remember to perform the lift-backs in a slow and consistent manner without jerking or overarching your lower back.

Rare is the complaint that our butts are too firm and tight. The following exercises are designed to push your butt muscles to the limit. By the way, do you remember what we told you

Quality Versus Quantity

Form (the quality of your efforts) is more important than frequency (the quantity or number of times you can repeat an exercise). It is more important to feel your muscles contracting with each repetition than racing to see how many you can do in one commercial break. Once you are sure of your form, you can start challenging yourself by attempting to do these exercises for the entire length of a commercial break.

about "spot-reducing"? Sorry, it still applies! The only way to get rid of unwanted body fat is through proper diet, proper caloric intake, and cardiovascular exercise. More about that later. For now, these exercises will strengthen your muscles, but they will not give you the buns of your dreams over night.

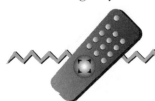

Exercise 2: Reclining Butt Crushers

DO THIS:

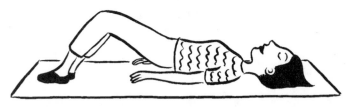

Hips lift off the floor by pushing down on heels; shoulders, upper back, and head stay on the floor

NOT THIS:

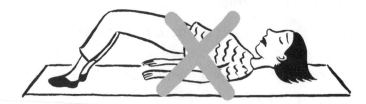

Hips pushed up so high that the back arches,
upper back off the floor, chin on the chest

1. Lie on your back with your knees bent and your feet flat on the floor. Inhale.

2. With your arms resting comfortably on the floor, exhale as you push down through the heels of your feet until your hips and butt come off the floor. Squeeze your butt muscles! Concentrate on keeping your upper back on the floor.

Suggested Program. Do reclining butt crushers through an entire commercial break.

Troubleshooting

Commercial Break

The next time you hear "You've Got Mail" on a television commercial, do a set of butt exercises. Keep the widening-butt monster away.

• Concentrate on feeling this primarily in your butt muscles (you will also feel it in your hamstrings a bit—this is okay).

• Be careful not to arch your back like a gymnast. You are doing butt lifts, not back bends.

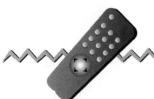

Exercise 3: One-Legged Butt Crushers

Wow! This exercise not only targets the butt, it also uses the hamstrings *and* the abdominal muscles for support as you balance. One-Legged Butt Crushers are similar to Exercise 2, with one big difference: These butt crushers are done one leg at a time.

1. Lie on the floor with your left knee bent and your left foot flat on the floor. Your right leg should be stretched out on the floor. Keep your arms comfortably on the floor next to you.

2. Lift your right leg about 6–8 inches off the floor. Inhale.

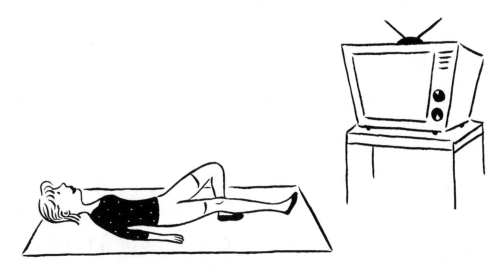

3. Exhale as you push down on your left foot, through the heel, until your butt and lower back come off the floor. Squeeze your butt muscles and hold for a count of 15 to 20. Breathe regularly through this exercise.

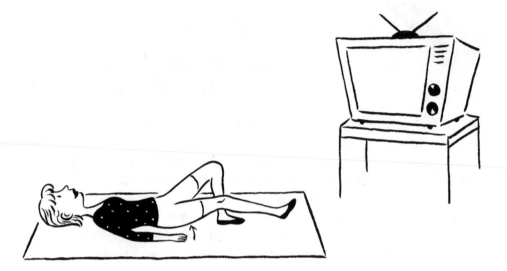

4. Inhale as you lower slowly.

5. Repeat this exercise through an entire product commercial.

6. Switch legs and repeat with the other leg for the next commercial.

Exercise 4: One-Legged Lunges

This more advanced exercise requires balance, abdominal strength, and good knowledge of proper knee position. If you have knee injuries or back problems, be cautious. We highly recommend that you use a sturdy chair to assist your balance while learning this one.

DO THIS:

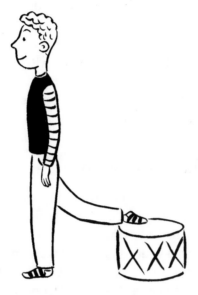

Head erect, shoulders back, chest open, knee stays over ankle, heel firmly on the floor

NOT THIS:

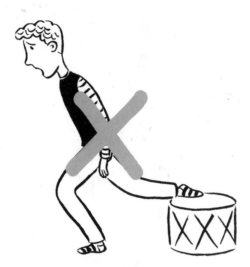

Chin dropped, shoulders rolled forward, back rounded, knee pushing past toes, heel off the floor

1. Get in a lunge position by placing your right leg behind you with the top of your right foot on the couch. If it's easier for you, you may also flex your foot so the ball of your foot is on the couch.

2. Balance on your left leg (use a sturdy chair to help with balance during the learning phase).

3. Inhale as you bend your left leg and lower your body so that your knee is at about 45 degrees. Make sure you can see your left toes at all times. Don't let the left knee go over the toes.

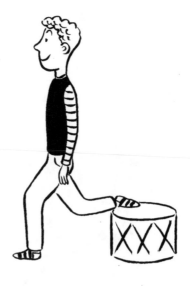

4. Exhale as you push through the heel on the floor to return to the starting position.

Suggested Program. Switch legs after each commercial spot. Do this exercise throughout an entire commercial break.

Troubleshooting

- Pain in the knees could mean many things. Be sure to check your body position and make sure your knee is not traveling over your toes. Remember to drop your back knee toward the floor as you bend your front knee. Keep your front shin perpendicular to the floor. If you continue to have knee discomfort, consult your physician.

- Discomfort in the lower back may be caused by poor posture. Be sure your head is neutral (not looking at the floor or ceiling). You should have a slight (natural) arch in your lower back, with your chest open, shoulders back, and abdominal muscles tight.

Gut

Remember high school gym class when someone held your feet while you strained and pulled to touch your knees with your chin? Aren't you glad fitness experts have decreed this method of abdominal work to not only be inefficient but also dangerous for your neck and back? Hurrah! Instead, cross your arms over your chest or *very lightly* support the back of your head with your *fingertips* (fingers should *not* be laced). Never, never, never pull on your neck. It is normal for your neck muscles to get tired (after all, the head weighs about 8 pounds). Don't worry, your neck and upper back muscles will get stronger with time.

The exercises in this section will strengthen your abdominal muscles—they will not locally remove fat. Remember, regardless of what many exercise equipment "infomercials" tell you, the only way to reduce body fat *anywhere* on your body is through proper diet and cardiovascular exercise. These subjects are discussed more completely in chapters 7 and 10.

"If 'crunches' don't burn the fat, then why bother?" you ask. Abdominal muscles are the "guy wires" that help stabilize the back. Strong abdominal muscles, along with the back muscles, are your central stabilizers. These muscles are known as your core. When there is weakness in this area, reduced stability, strength, and function are often the result. Abdominal muscles allow you to do simple tasks, such as tying your shoes, and more complex endeavors, such as balancing a water bottle on a sandwich plate as you search for the TV remote!

Again, the exercises in this section start out simple and become more difficult and complex as you go. Do not move on to the next level of exercise until you feel comfortable with the current exercise.

Exercise 5: Crunches

DO THIS:

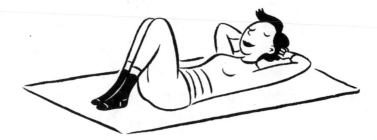

Head neutral, shoulders and upper back come off the floor,
lower and middle back press against the floor

NOT THIS:

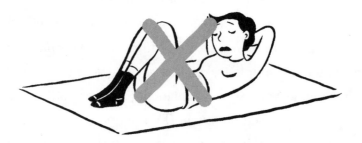

Chin resting on chest, fingers laced behind head/neck, back arched

1. Lie on your back with your knees bent, feet flat on the floor.

2. Make fists with your hands and place your knuckles against
   the side of your head, or place your fingertips along your head
   and neck. Don't lace your fingers together. Your hands are
   there for support, not to lift your head.

3. Your head must stay in a neutral position throughout this exercise. In other words, your neck will be straight. Don't tuck your chin or point your chin to the ceiling, just look straight ahead. Inhale.

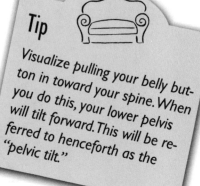

Tip

Visualize pulling your belly button in toward your spine. When you do this, your lower pelvis will tilt forward. This will be referred to henceforth as the "pelvic tilt."

4. Exhale while pressing your lower back against the floor. This will raise your upper torso slightly.

5. Hold this position for a count of 3. You will feel the muscles around your middle tighten. Only your head, neck, shoulders, and upper back will be off the floor.

6. Keep your abdominal muscles tight as you inhale and lower yourself slowly back to the floor.

Suggested Program. Repeat for at least one commercial. As you get stronger, add commercials until you can do this exercise for an entire commercial break.

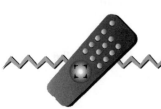

Exercise 6:
Elevated-Leg Crunches

When it comes to your body, variety is the key to change. If the regular crunch gets too easy, mix it up a bit by doing crunches with your feet elevated.

1. Lie on your back with your feet resting on the seat of a chair, sofa, or hassock. Your knees should be perpendicular to the hips, not over your chest. Inhale.

2. Make fists with your hands, place them against the side of your head, and keep your head neutral. Exhale as you curl your chest and shoulders toward your knees.

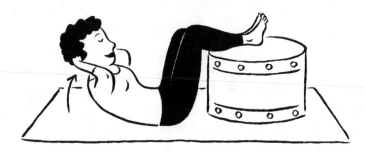

Challenging Option. If this becomes too easy, forgo using the footrest. Instead, perform the crunch with your feet unsupported and your legs elevated over your hips. Keep your knees relaxed and your back flat on the floor.

Troubleshooting

- It is only necessary to lift about 6 inches off the floor.

- Remember to keep your lower back (tailbone) flat against the floor by tilting your pelvis.

- Your shoulders and upper back are the only parts of your body that come off the floor. Keep the lower and mid-back on the floor.

Commercial Break

The next time you see an ad that shows people walking around in skimpy bathing suits, do a set of abdominal exercises.

Exercise 7: Roll-Up Crunches

DO THIS:

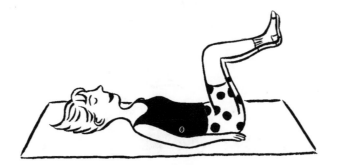

Lower back flat on floor, knees come to chest by
contracting abdominal muscles

NOT THIS:

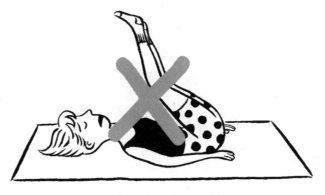

Lower back arched, legs flung wildly over torso

1. Lie on the floor with your knees bent and your feet on the floor. The backs of your arms should be resting on the floor, with your hands either under your tailbone or flat on the floor, whichever is most comfortable. Inhale.

2. Exhale while pressing your lower back to the floor and, without using your hands, pulling your knees as close as you can to your chest/chin. Your lower back should remain on the floor. Avoid any rocking of your hips and lower back.

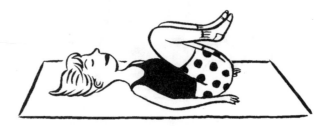

3. Tighten your "gut" as hard as you can without holding your breath. Relax this muscle slowly and inhale while lowering your legs back to the starting position.

Suggested Program. Repeat the Roll-Up Crunches as many times as you can during one commercial break.

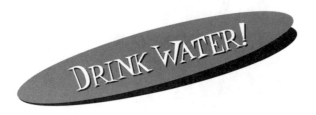

Exercise 8: Challenging Crunches

This particular crunch will give your routine a bit more variety.

1. Start from a sitting position on the floor, with your feet flat on the floor and knees bent in front of you. Inhale.

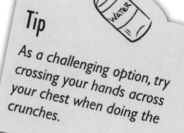

Tip

As a challenging option, try crossing your hands across your chest when doing the crunches.

2. Keeping your back curved and your head neutral, exhale as you slowly lower your body, vertebrae by vertebrae, to the floor.

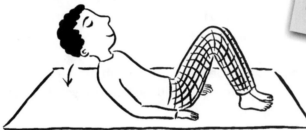

3. When your back is all the way to the floor, lift one leg and use the momentum of putting it *back* on the floor to roll you back up to the start position.

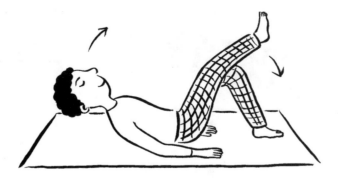

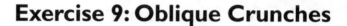

Exercise 9: Oblique Crunches

Have you ever had a secret desire to be a hula dancer? Want to win the next "Bump" contest at "Remember-the-Seventies Night"? Strengthening the quatratus lumborum (a muscle of the lower back that is attached to the posterior side of the pelvis), also known as the "hip hiker," is your answer. This exercise will take the snaggle out of your waggle and can help you master that wiggle as well!

1. Lie on your right side. Support your upper torso with your right elbow/forearm and your left hand. Your left leg will be lying on top of your right leg. Keep your legs relaxed. Do not lock your knees. Inhale.

2. Exhale as you lift both legs as a unit about 4–6 inches off the ground. Angle your legs slightly in front of you (rolling onto your butt slightly).

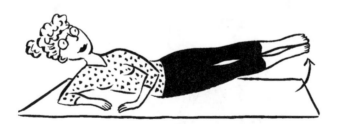

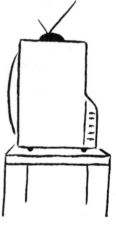

3. Return your legs to the start position and repeat for one product advertisement.

4. Repeat on your left side.

Challenging Option. Cross your arms over your chest and try lifting your upper torso at the same time that you lift your lower torso!

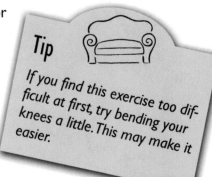

Tip

If you find this exercise too difficult at first, try bending your knees a little. This may make it easier.

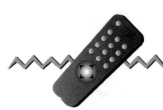

Exercise 10: Bicycles

This exercise is an oldie but a goodie! Bicycles are a great exercise for the entire abdominal muscle group.

1. Lie on your back with your feet off the floor, knees over your hips. Your fingertips will be supporting your head, which will remain in the neutral position throughout the exercise, even when turning from side to side.

2. Move your legs as if you were riding a bicycle. As a knee comes toward your chest, turn your torso so the opposite elbow and shoulder reaches toward it. Perform this exercise slooooowly for best results!

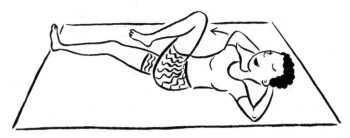

3. Be sure to breathe!

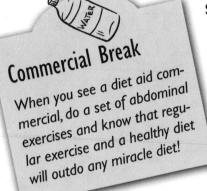

Commercial Break

When you see a diet aid commercial, do a set of abdominal exercises and know that regular exercise and a healthy diet will outdo any miracle diet!

Suggested Program. Try to do this exercise for an entire commercial break. When you finish with your crunches, stretch your abdominal muscles and lower back (see chapter 3, stretch 17).

Exercise 11: Crossover Crunches

Here is another, more difficult exercise for the oblique muscles, which are located on each side of your abdomen beneath the "love handles." When Crossover Crunches are done correctly (which is a euphemism for "this is a whole lot harder than it looks"), you will definitely feel tighter and stronger around your waist.

DO THIS:

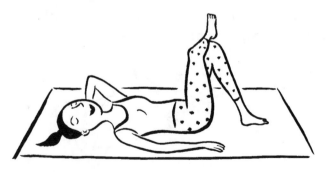

Right ankle resting just above left knee, fingertips of left hand supporting head, right arm resting on floor, left elbow remains out of your peripheral, head and eyes stay focused on opposite knee

NOT THIS:

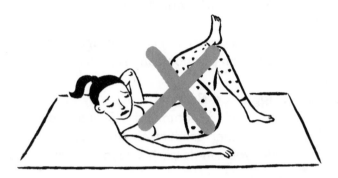

Head turned so eyes are on floor, arm behind head coming across
body, knees coming across as they try to touch on the diagonal,
head being pulled off neutral by arm

1. Lie on your back with your left leg bent and your left foot flat
   on the floor. Your right ankle is on your left knee, right arm
   resting on the floor, and left arm supporting your head. Inhale.

2. Without allowing your right knee or your left elbow to move
   toward each other, exhale as you lift your left shoulder toward your right knee. Keep your elbow back.

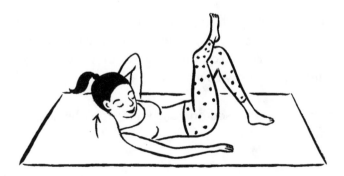

3. Keep your eyes on your right knee as you lift your shoulder toward it. If you can see your left elbow, you are doing
   it wrong!

Remember

Everyone has different levels of mobility. When doing crunches, lift your shoulder as far as you can while keeping the middle of your back on the floor.

4. You should feel this in the area of your oblique muscles (below the ribs).

5. After finishing a set on the right side, switch leg and arm positions, and repeat for the left side.

Suggested Program. Start by doing one side for one product commercial. Switch sides and repeat for another product commercial. Add commercials until you can do each side for an entire commercial break.

Troubleshooting

- "Less is more." Your shoulder may be just an inch or two off the floor.

- Are you keeping your elbow and knee from coming toward each other? Do not "collapse" your elbow or allow your knee to pull in toward the elbow.

- Are you lifting your shoulder toward your knee? (*Note:* You will not be able to actually touch your shoulder to your knee!) You should be rotating your shoulder toward your knee, not your elbow toward your knee.

- Keep your eyes focused on your knee; don't let them wander off toward the floor.

Have you noticed that all of the exercises in the book so far are for strengthening the major muscle groups? Perhaps you are gleefully hoping that we left out the dreaded "huffy puffy" stuff? Not so. Please turn to chapter 7 during the next commercial break to get started on the all-important cardiovascular (heart/ lung) exercises. We put these exercises in their own chapter so that we could fully explain the importance of "huffing and puffing" for your overall health.

Tip

After doing the exercises in this chapter, it is a good idea to do the chest and lower back stretches in chapter 3 (particularly Stretches 1 through 8).

chapter seven

Ya Gotta Have Heart!

Media attention on heart disease has traditionally focused on men, leading many women to believe that they shouldn't be concerned with heart disease. Breast cancer, which has a higher media profile, is sometimes assumed to be more dangerous to women than heart disease. But it ain't necessarily so! Statistics show that heart disease kills five times more women than does breast cancer. Then why aren't women dashing about in a jogging frenzy, huffing and puffing their way to heart health?

We often hear the voice of defeat when it comes to cardio-vascular exercise. Simply with regular exercise, both women and men could improve their odds against heart disease and other metabolic disorders associated with a sedentary lifestyle. In fact, according to the Web site www.ridinactivity.org, if the average adult would walk an additional 600 feet a day over a 10-year period, 10 pounds of fat could be avoided!

Before we get into the actual "huffy puffy" exercises designed to start you on a healthful heart and lung program, let's set the "Way-Back Machine" for junior-high health class and revisit the basics of the cardiovascular system.

"Blood pressure," "cholesterol," "LDL," "HDL," "triglycerides" . . . these terms are bandied about from tête-à-tête to talk show. But what do they all mean? Since almost everyone has had his or her arm constricted by a blood pressure cuff at some time or another, let's start with blood pressure.

Blood Pressure and Hypertension

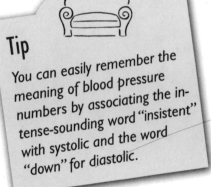

Tip
You can easily remember the meaning of blood pressure numbers by associating the intense-sounding word "insistent" with systolic and the word "down" for diastolic.

Blood pressure is the force that flowing blood exerts against the walls of the arteries. The pressure exerted against the arterial walls when the heart contracts, or beats, is the top number of your blood pressure reading (systolic pressure). The second number of your blood pressure reading represents the pressure exerted against the arterial wall when the heart rests between beats (diastolic pressure). Generally, a blood pressure reading of 120/80 is considered optimal, with normal at 130/85. What is normal for *you*, however, will depend on your age, gender, and family history.

Hypertension is a condition generally indicated by a systolic pressure reading of 140 and above and a diastolic pressure of 90 and above. Again, this should be adjusted for gender and age. Your doctor or medical professional is the best person to properly evaluate your blood pressure reading for you. Hypertension is dangerous because it increases the risk for stroke, heart failure, kidney disease, and aneurysm.

The risk factors for hypertension are:

1. The foods you eat (dietary)

2. How physically active you are (sedentary lifestyle)

3. If you are a smoker (or live with one)

4. Your genetic predisposition (hereditary)

5. Whether you live with a teenager (stress!)

As grim as all of this may seem, the easiest and most natural way to control hypertension is . . . (drum roll) . . . regular cardiovascular exercise. *Cardiovascular* refers to the heart (*cardio*) and the blood vessels (*vascular*) as a unified system in the body. The heart is a muscle. Like all muscles in the body, the heart needs to be conditioned to stay healthy and strong. By exercising the heart, the blood vessels are exercised as well, which helps them keep their integrity. Cardiovascular exercise also helps prevent blood vessels from becoming brittle and/or clogged with fatty goo acquired from consistently eating foods that are high in *cholesterol* (how's that for a slick segue into our next topic?).

Cholesterol and Triglycerides

So, what is this cholesterol stuff, anyhow? Why are we told to avoid it?

Cholesterol, which is produced in the liver, is an odorless, waxy substance that travels around the body via the bloodstream. In spite of the fact that cholesterol is found in *all* foods of animal origin, it cannot be tasted or seen. Our body uses cholesterol to make essential substances, such as the lining of our cell walls. Although the main source of blood cholesterol is produced by our liver, studies indicate that a couch-potato lifestyle high in the consumption of animal products (meat, cheese, whole milk, cream) and low in fruits, vegetables, grains, and beans can elevate blood cholesterol to the degree that it no longer passes easily through the blood vessels. Instead, it sticks to the sides and starts to build up . . . like the sludge on a kitchen pipe (yuck!).

To understand your cardiac risk level, you must know the ratio between "good" and "bad" cholesterol, or HDL and LDL, respectively. Because cholesterol is a fat and not water-soluble, it must combine with proteins in the blood so that it can be used by the body. When cholesterol, blood proteins, and fats combine in the blood, the substance is referred to as lipoprotein. If you eat plenty of lowfat, high-fiber foods, your cholesterol will become high-density lipoprotein (HDL). Because HDL particles are small and dense, they do not stick to the wall of your arteries. This type of cholesterol is known as "good" cholesterol. Think of HDL cholesterol as little scouring pads that take the sludge in your blood to your liver for removal.

The flip side of HDL cholesterol is LDL and VLDL cholesterol. LDL (low-density lipoproteins) and VLDL (very low-density lipoproteins) are the sludge, or the "bad" cholesterol. These two types of cholesterol deposit fat along artery walls. To increase your good cholesterol and reduce your bad, it's recommended that you do the following:

1. Engage in regular exercise.

2. Do not smoke.

3. Eat a high-fiber diet (including lots of fruits, vegetables, grains, and beans) that is also low in saturated fat.

4. Reduce stresses.

That's the good and the bad. Now for the ugly—triglycerides. Ninety-five percent of the total fats stored in the body are triglycerides. Their main job is to provide you with energy. When not used, triglycerides are stored in fat cells, which are situated throughout the body, often around your organs. A high triglyceride level often coincides with a low HDL and a high LDL blood profile. It is often found in heavy drinkers of alcohol, smokers, the obese, and the sedentary. The three fatty acids that comprise the triglyceride molecule are all highly saturated, which increases the risk for coronary heart disease when levels are too high in the blood.

Cholesterol and triglycerides are measured in the blood as milligrams per deciliter (mg/dl). The National Institute of Health recommends the following general guidelines as a healthy standard:

Total cholesterol: Between 120–200 mg/dl

HDL cholesterol: Between 35–65 mg/dl (it should also account for more than 25 percent of total cholesterol)

LDL cholesterol: Between 60–160 mg/dl

Triglycerides: Between 10–160 mg/dl

Note: For best results, your doctor should measure your cholesterol levels by using the average of three tests from a full blood draw, known as your "ratio," rather than a total count assessed through just one finger prick.

Coronary Risk Ratio

Blood pressure readings, cholesterol levels, HDL/LDL ratios, and triglyceride levels are a few of the various factors used to determine your coronary risk ratio. Your particular coronary risk ratio is also determined by a variety of factors that are unique to you, such as your activity level, smoking history, amount of stress, and genetics. We strongly recommend an annual physical exam by a qualified health-care professional. The general information in this chapter is to be used only as a guide, so that you can better discuss coronary risk factors with your physician.

Calculating Exercise Intensity

You may have noticed the "E" word popping up frequently in our discussion of cardiovascular health! The rest of this chapter outlines a basic program designed to give you a feel for cardiovascular *exercise*. Our objective is to get you started on a cardiovascular exercise regimen that you can do while enjoying your favorite television programs. These exercises will stimulate your heart muscle and increase your rate of breathing. *Proceed slowly*.

If you are new to cardiovascular exercise, or if you have been away from regular exercise for a while, it is important to be aware of your exertion level. We have included a scale that will allow you to easily measure (perceive) your level of exertion. This scale is known as the Borg Scale for Perceived Exertion. (No, this is *not* "the Borg" from "Star Trek" . . . resistance is *not* futile, and you will *not* be assimilated.)

Perceived exertion means you have to pay attention to how you are feeling. This will come in handy as you push yourself harder in your workout. If you perceive that you are working *very* hard, and if this is uncomfortable for you, reduce your level of intensity or return to the previous level. For example, if you are doing Quick Steps (Exercise 3) and feel that you are working very, very hard and are not comfortable with the intensity, slow your pace. The numbers on the scale correlate to what you perceive your intensity to be. By adding a zero to the end of these numbers, they correlate to a range of heart-rate intensities. For example, 6 = 60 and 12 = 120:

The Borg Scale

The Borg Scale was developed by Gunnar Borg, Ph.D., professor emeritus at the University of Stockholm, Sweden. What made Borg's study revolutionary was that he used human perception, rather than mechanical technology, as a scientific instrument to determine exertion levels.

Borg Scale of Perceived Exertion

6	7	8	9	10	11	12	13	14	15	16	17	18	19	20

very, very light	fairly light	hard	very hard	extremely hard
(beginner)	(moderate)	(advanced)	(intense—not recommended)	

Another indicator of too much exertion is when you cannot say a whole string of words, such as "Mary had a little lamb," without taking a breath. If you can't say this simple statement, then you are at your maximum level. We do *not* recommend that you exercise at your maximum exertion level. Instead, you should strive to exercise in the 50–80 percent range of what *you perceive* to be your maximum.

We recommend that you begin by exercising at *your* comfort level, wherever that is. You will begin to feel warm all over as you do the exercises. *Slow down* or *stop* if you feel out of breath, if you cannot talk comfortably or feel lightheaded while exercising.

Enough procrastinating—onward and forward!

Maximum Heart Rate

To compute your maximum heart rate/exercise intensity, subtract your age from 220 (the number of beats per minute regarded by experts as the heart's predicted maximum) and multiply by a number between .50 and .80, which represents your desired intensity. For example, if you are 45 years old and want to work out at 60 percent of your maximum intensity, do the following computation:

$220 - 45 = 175 \times .60 = 105$, or 10.5 on the Borg Scale.

Get Ready . . .

For those of you who consider it "cardiovascular exercise" when you dash from the couch to the bathroom and then to the refrigerator, we recommend that you start at the Beginning Level. Since you do not want to miss any part of the show that you are watching, we suggest that you do the following during the first few commercials:

1. Replace the soda, beer, or juice with *water*.

2. Visit the john.

3. Be sure that you are wearing comfortable, supportive athletic shoes and clothing.

4. Have a towel handy.

5. Clear the floor of TV guides, remote control devices, cat toys, dog bones, sharp-edged tables, and so forth.

Remember your posture—maintain proper alignment, tighten your abdominal muscles, and keep your head neutral. Relax your shoulders.

When you're finished exercising, "cool down" before flopping back down on the couch. Walk around for a minute or two to allow your heart rate to return to normal and to keep your muscles from cramping. This is a good plan to follow regardless of your fitness level. It is necessary to cool down after every workout, no matter the intensity or duration. Your muscles,

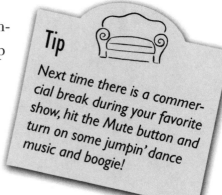

Tip

Next time there is a commercial break during your favorite show, hit the Mute button and turn on some jumpin' dance music and boogie!

DRINK WATER!

as well as your cardiovascular and respiratory systems, need to recuperate. You should also stretch after any type of exercise. Stretching when your muscles are lubricated and warm helps increase flexibility and reduce soreness.

Cardiovascular Exercise Tips

• It is important to start any cardiovascular workout with a 3 to 5 minute warm-up and to end it with a 3 to 5 minute cool-down.

• Drink 8 to 10 ounces of water for every hour of your workout.

• Pay close attention to your level of exertion and how it feels to you. If you cannot speak in normal sentences while exercising, slow down.

• Be aware of your posture and body alignment.

• Most important: *Have fun!*

Get Set ...

Warm Up

Simply stand by your easy chair and march gently in place, swinging your arms in a controlled manner, elbows slightly bent. Your feet should barely leave the floor. Stop when your show resumes. Drink some water and relax.

Go!

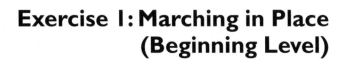

Exercise 1: Marching in Place
(Beginning Level)

1. As you did during your warm-up, stand by your chair and march in place, but this time keep marching for two to three commercials.

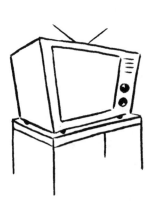
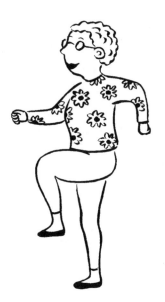

2. If you feel like doing something a bit more challenging, lift your knees higher as you march, and swing your arms a bit more. Keep those abdominal muscles tight. Your objective is to bring the top of your knee to a right angle (90-degree angle) with your hips. Your knee will be bent at the same right angle.

3. Repeat this routine for every commercial during the first 30 minutes of your television program.

Initial Goal. Do this routine for every commercial break during 2 hours of TV programming. Check your perceived exertion on the Borg Scale. Try to increase your level of intensity.

Ultimate Goal. Perform this exercise during the entire TV program, *resting* during commercials.

Challenging Option. As you place your feet on the floor, alternate back and forth between a narrow marching stance to a wide "walking-in-tires" stance (simply move your feet farther apart as if each foot were in the center of a big rubber tire). This will give your legs and butt a bit more attention.

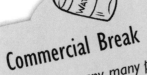

Commercial Break

There are many, many prescription drug advertisements on TV. Take advantage of these 30-second breaks to do some cardiovascular work and keep your heart healthy!

Once you feel as if you are in the 6–8 range of the Borg Scale doing this more challenging option, it is time to proceed to the Moderate Level.

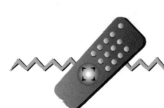

Exercise 2: Ice Skater's Move (Moderate Level)

Congratulations! This jump to the next level means that your heart muscle is getting stronger.

1. Before beginning this exercise, warm up by marching in place for one commercial.

2. As the second commercial begins, increase the intensity by stepping from side to side as if you were an ice skater: Right leg steps to the right and is joined by the left leg, then left leg steps back to the original position and is rejoined by the right leg.

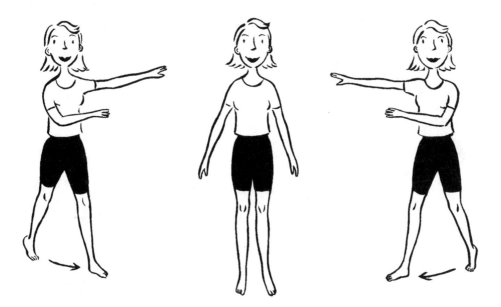

3. Allow your arms to swing naturally along with the movement.

4. Repeat as many times as you can for the remainder of the commercial break.

Initial Goal. Perform this exercise for every commercial break during 2 consecutive hours of TV programming.

Ultimate Goal. Do this exercise during the entire TV program. Rest during the commercials.

Check your perceived exertion on the Borg Scale. You should feel like you are in the 9–12 range, which would be like working at about 70 percent of your predicted maximum. Always use your best judgment and challenge yourself when you feel you are ready to do so.

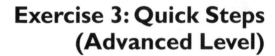

Remember that when exercising, you must maintain good posture: head neutral, abdominal muscles tight, shoulders relaxed. After exercising, it is important to cool down slightly before getting back to your couch. Walk to the kitchen and get some water to drink, or walk around for 2 to 5 minutes before sitting or reclining.

Once your perceived exertion level is 9–12, move on to the Advanced Level.

Exercise 3: Quick Steps (Advanced Level)

Wow! Your fitness level has *really* improved! You definitely "have heart." For the first commercial, do the warm-up. For the rest of the commercial break, switch to the Moderate Level (Ice Skater's Move). At the second commercial break, start the Quick Steps.

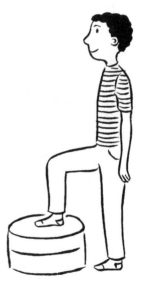

1. Find a step, bench, stair, or footstool that is about 6–8 inches high. Make sure it is secure so that there is no chance of it slipping out from under you.

2. Starting with your right leg, step up onto the step/stair/bench/footstool with your entire foot, allowing the heel of the foot to strike first.

3. Bring the left foot up to join the right foot on the step.

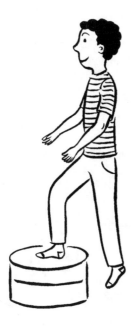
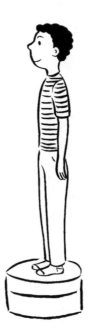

4. Step back down to the floor, right foot first, followed by the left foot.

5. Continue leading with the right foot for the rest of the commercial break.

6. At the next commercial break, lead with the left foot. Your arms should be at your side, swinging normally.

Challenging Option. Lift your arms overhead for the step up. Bring them back to shoulder level for the step down. Continue this pattern for the entire commercial break.

Initial Goal. Do this exercise at every commercial break for 2 hours of TV programming.

Ultimate Goal. Perform this exercise during the entire TV program and *rest* during the commercials.

chapter **8** eight

Time to Exercise

Because No One Wants to Be the Weakest Link!

The TV is on. You have your water at the ready. You have a copy of this book sitting next to you. And you are finally ready to put it all together and start exercising. What do you do first? Which exercises should you try during the next commercial break? In spite of having everything right at your fingertips, it is sometimes still hard to get going. So, to eliminate the inevitable inertia, here are some sample programs to get you going on the path to a healthier you.

We have included six programs of exercise in this chapter. There are two beginner programs, two intermediate, and two advanced.

Beginning at the Beginning

We'll start with two easy programs for the person who has not exercised since the Earth's crust cooled, or at least in a long, long while. These are suggested time frames only. If you feel you need more time and want to spread your workout over more commercial breaks, by all means do so. These exercises are designed to be accomplished during 2 to 3 hours of TV, give or take a "sitcom."

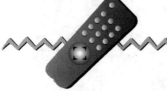

Program 1

After getting your water, donning comfortable clothing, and locating the remote and the TV schedule, proceed with Program 1!

Commercial Break 1

- Stand by your chair with your eyes closed and practice the Easy Balance Exercise (page 16). Do this through two product commercials.

- For the rest of the commercial break, warm up by Marching in Place (page 123).

Commercial Break 2

- The stretch for Neck Flexibility (page 24) should feel good about now! Do this stretch for one product commercial.

- During the second product spot, stretch the Upper Back and Shoulders (page 27).

- For the third commercial, perform the "Cat" Stretch (page 31).

- And finally, for the fourth commercial, stretch with the Back Curve (page 33).

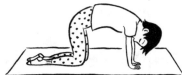

Commercial Break 3

For this break, you have your choice of either Isometrics (page 45) or Wall Pushups (page 46). Since you will be doing this for an entire commercial break, you may want to alternate between the two. Simply change exercises as the commercials change.

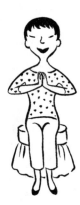

Commercial Break 4

- Do Chair Squats (page 70) for as many commercials as you can. Your ultimate goal is to perform this exercise for an entire commercial break. But start slowly, and make sure you concentrate on proper form.

- Follow the Chair Squats with some stretches for the hips, butt, and legs (pages 34–37) during the remaining commercials in the break.

- Finish up by doing some Toe Taps (page 84) for the first few minutes of the television program.

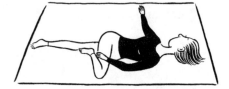

Commercial Break 5

- Do the Butt Lift-Backs (page 90) for an entire commercial break. Switch legs after each product advertisement.

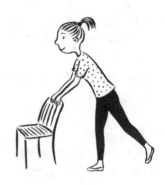

Commercial Break 6

- Time for Crunches (page 100)! Perform as many of these as you can for the entire commercial break.

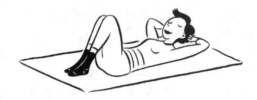

Commercial Break 7

- Marching in Place (page 123) is a great way to finish your exercise session.

Commercial Break 8

But wait! There's more! The show is not over yet. There's one more commercial break. It's the perfect time to stretch!

Do each of the following stretches for a different product commercial.

- Neck and Spine (page 25)

- Upper Back and Shoulders with a Twist (page 28)

- Leg Pull (page 32)

Finish up with some Relaxed Breathing (page 20).

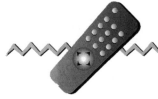

Program 2

Here's another "Ease-Into-This-Healthy-Stuff-Gradually" program.

Commercial Break 1

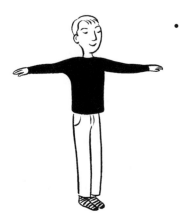

- Stand by your chair with your eyes closed and practice the Easy Balance Exercise (page 16). Do this for an entire commercial break. Be sure to check your posture during at least one of the commercial spots.

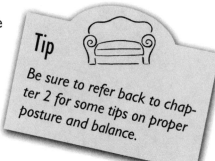

Tip

Be sure to refer back to chapter 2 for some tips on proper posture and balance.

Commercial Break 2

- Warm up by Marching in Place (page 123) for the entire commercial break. Or better yet, march to the laundry room, bathroom, or kitchen (be sure to grab some water!).

Commercial Break 3

For the third commercial break, do a couple stretches.

- Start with the Neck and Spine stretch (page 25).

- For the next commercial, get down on the floor for Reclining Neck Rolls (page 26).

- While you are on the floor, do the Upper Body Stretch (page 30).

- Finish up the commercial break with the Leg Pull (page 32).

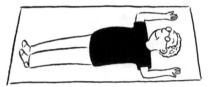

Commercial Break 4

- Do Wall Pushups for chest (page 46) for an entire commercial break.

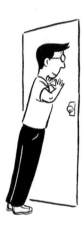

Commercial Break 5

- Start the commercial break by doing Triceps Wall Pushups (page 59) for at least three commercials.

- Next lie face down on the floor for The "X" back strengthener (page 57).

- Perform Superman (page 58) for the rest of the break.

Commercial Break 6

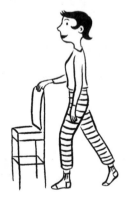

- Your legs will love Pulsing Lunges (page 73). Pay attention to your form and don't rush this exercise.

- Switch legs for each product spot, or after 10 to 12 pulses with each leg.

Commercial Break 7

- Do Reclining Butt Crushers (page 93) for an entire commercial break.

- During the first minute of the TV program, perform Basic Calf Raises (page 85).

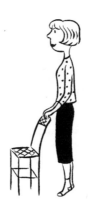

Commercial Break 8

For this break, you'll be alternating between two types of exercise as the commercials change.

- For the first commercial, do Crunches (page 100).

- For the second commercial, do some Roll-Up Crunches (page 103).

- For the third commercial, go back to the Crunches. And so on and so forth until its time to get back to your regularly scheduled programming.

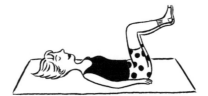

Commercial Break 9

Here's another combination set. Alternate exercises for each new commercial.

- For the first commercial, do some Marching in Place (page 123).

Tip

Remember to use the Borg Scale to monitor your perceived exertion level (see the chart on page 120).

- For the next commercial, perform the Ice Skater's Move (page 124).

- Another option is to switch between the two exercises during the 30-second commercials—15 seconds of marching; 15 seconds of skating!

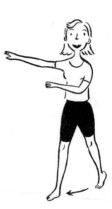

Commercial Break 10

Finish your exercise program by relaxing with your favorite stretches, such as the Neck and Spine stretch (page 25) and the Abdominal stretch (page 40).

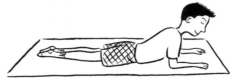

Intermediate Programs

For those of you who have successfully mastered the previous program suggestions (or a reasonable facsimile thereof), you are probably ready for more of a push. Try these!

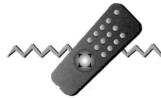

Program 3

With TV schedule and remote in hand (or on a table), you are ready to test yourself with some more difficult exercises and combinations. As we mentioned before, these timeframes are suggestions only and are not meant to be etched into stone (or even last year's fruitcake).

Commercial Break 1

Before you start exercising, stand in front of the TV and do a quick posture check. Is your head in alignment with your spine? Are your shoulders down and relaxed? If you need a reminder, go to page 13 and review the good posture illustration.

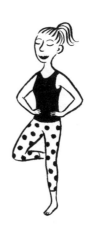

- Start off with some more balance work. The Flamingo (page 18) is perfect for this. Hold each one-legged pose for an entire product commercial. Switch ONLY between products.

Commercial Break 2

DRINK WATER!

- Warm up with some Marching in Place (page 123), mixed with some Ice Skater's Move (page 124) for the entire commercial break.

Commercial Break 3

- For the first commercial, start with some Upper Back and Shoulders with a Twist stretches (page 28).

- For commercial number two, move on to the Upper Back Slide (page 29).

- Next, roll onto your back to perform the stretch for Hips and Butt (page 34).

Remember

If you feel you need more time, spread these stretches out over two commercial breaks.

- During the third commercial, stretch the Chest (page 38).

- Finish off with some stretches for the Triceps (page 39).

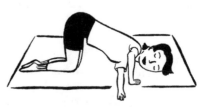

Commercial Break 4

- Warm up for one commercial with the All-Fours Pushups (page 48).

- As soon as the next commercial starts, go right into Knee Pushups (page 50).

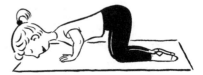

Commercial Break 5

- Warm up your back muscles with The "X" (page 57) for one commercial.

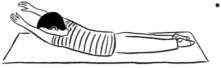

- For the next commercial, do Superman (page 58). Alternate between lifting arms and then legs with each commercial spot for the rest of the commercial break.

Commercial Break 6

- Perform the Triceps Wall Pushups (page 59) for an entire commercial break.

Commercial Break 7

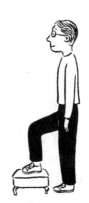

- Warm up your legs by doing Chair Squats (page 70) for one commercial.

- Then proceed to Step-Ups (page 77) for the remainder of the commercials in that break.

Commercial Break 8

- Warm up by doing Reclining Butt Crushers (page 93) for one commercial.

- For the rest of the commercials of this break, do One-Legged Butt Crushers (page 95).

- For the first few minutes of the TV program, perform Basic Calf Raises (page 85).

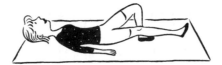

Commercial Break 9

Alternate between three different crunches for the entire commercial break, switching between each crunch for each different product advertised.

- Crunches (page 100)

- Roll-Up Crunches (page 103)

- Oblique Crunches (page 106)

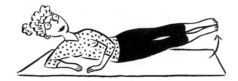

Tip

Keep the Borg Scale handy (see the table on page 120) to check your exertion level. Take note of your Active Breathing patterns (see page 20).

Commercial Breaks 10 and 11

It's time to work that heart muscle!

- Do both the Marching in Place and the Ice Skater's Move. Alternate between the two with every other commercial.

Commercial Break 12

And what do you end with? Stretches, of course! Try some of these stretches for each commercial:

- Hamstrings (page 35)

- Quadriceps (page 36)

- The "Butterfly" (page 37)

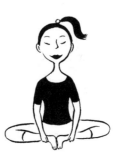

Finish with an Abdominal stretch (page 40) and the Waist Twist (page 41).

Another Intermediate Level Program

Program 4

For variety and to avoid boredom, we suggest that you move on to something a little more challenging. Try this one on for size.

Commercial Break 1

- Work on the Flamingo balancing exercise (page 18). Switch from leg to leg as product commercials change during the break.

- If that gets too easy, try to stand without holding on to anything.

- If you are feeling really adventurous, try this balance pose with your eyes closed!

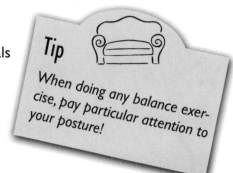

Tip

When doing any balance exercise, pay particular attention to your posture!

Commercial Break 2

- Warm up with some Marching in Place (page 123).

- Mix in some Ice Skater's Move (page 124).

- Alternate between Marching in Place and the Ice Skater's Move for the entire commercial break.

Tip

Be sure to use your arms to give yourself a good total body warm-up. Arms also help with balance!

Commercial Break 3

- Start with the "Cat" Stretch (page 31).

- From the "Cat" Stretch, push yourself up into the Back Curve (page 33).

- Then proceed with a stretch for the Hips and Butt (page 34).

- Next stretch out the Hamstrings (page 35). You can also add the optional feet, ankle, and calf stretch this time.

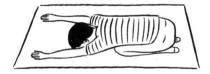

Commercial Break 4

- Do Knee Pushups (page 50) for one commercial.

- For the rest of the commercial break, try Elevated Pushups (page 52).

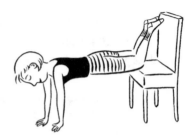

Commercial Break 5

- Do the Superman back strengthener (page 58) for the first two product advertisements (switching from lifting arms to lifting legs for each commercial).

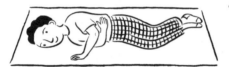

- For the next commercial, go right into Single-Arm Triceps Pushups (page 61). Switch between left and right arms with each product advertised.

Commercial Break 6

- Warm up your legs with Step-Ups (page 77) for one commercial.

- For the remainder of the commercials, perform the Sumo Squats (page 78).

- Before sitting down again, be sure to repeat the leg stretches performed earlier during Commecial Break 3.

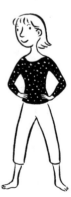

Commercial Break 7

- Continue your leg workout by performing Hamstring Pulses (page 82). Switch legs for each product advertised.

- After four commercials, switch to One-Legged Butt Crushers (page 95). If there are enough commercials left, switch legs for each product advertised.

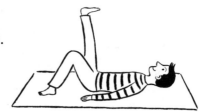

Commercial Break 8

- Warm up with basic Crunches (page 100) for an entire commercial.

- For the rest of the commercials, switch between Roll-Up Crunches (page 103) and Challenging Crunches (page 105).

Commercial Break 9

For this commercial break, alternate among the following three abdominal exercises:

- Oblique Crunches (page 106)

- Bicycles (page 107)

- Crossover Crunches (page 108)

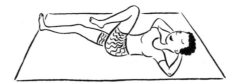

Commercial Break 10

It is time for the huffy-puffys!

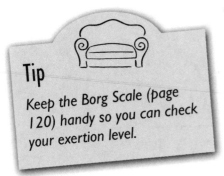

Tip

Keep the Borg Scale (page 120) handy so you can check your exertion level.

- Do both the Marching in Place (page 123) and the Ice Skater's Move (page 124). Alternate between the two every other commercial.

- This might be a good time to walk up and down the stairs once or twice or march from room to room.

- Before sitting down, cool down with some slow Marching in Place until your Perceived Exertion Level is at about 7.

Commercial Break 11

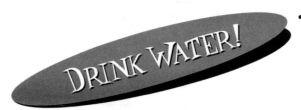

- Repeat the stretches performed earlier in this program. You can add in any of your favorite stretches.

- Practice some Relaxed Breathing (page 20) before sitting back to enjoy the rest of your TV show.

Advanced Programs

If you have been working with our program consistently and are prepared to try even more challenges, get ready for a top-notch workout!

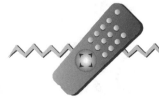

Program 5

Commercial Break 1

Before you begin the exercises, stand in front of a mirror and check your posture. Look at the illustration on page 13 to be sure you are in proper alignment.

- Warm up with the Flamingo balancing exercise (page 18).

- For the next commercial, perform the Hardest Balance Exercise (page 19).

Tip

For both balancing exercises in Break 1, try the "Look ma, no hands" version for an extra challenge.

Commercial Break 2

- Warm up by Marching in Place (page 123) and performing the Ice Skater's Move (page 124) for two commercials.

- For the remaining commercials, do Quick Steps (page 126). Pay close attention to your heart rate and perceived exertion before sitting down at the end of the break. Make sure that you are breathing normally and that you don't feel too overexerted.

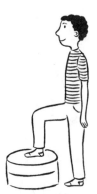

Commercial Break 3

- Start with the Neck and Spine stretch (page 25) for one commercial.

- For the second commercial, move on to the Upper Back and Shoulders stretch (page 27).

- During the third commercial, do the Upper Back Slide (page 29).

- Finish off the commercial break with the Upper Body Stretch (page 30).

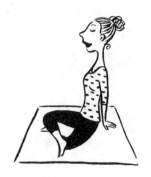

Commercial Break 4

For each commercial, perform you favorite leg stretches. Choose from any of the following:

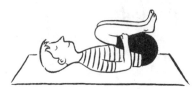

- Leg Pull (page 32)

- Hamstrings (page 35)

- Quadriceps (page 36)

If there is still one more commercial to go in this break, finish with the Chest (page 38) and Triceps (page 39).

Commercial Break 5

- Warm up with Elevated Pushups (page 52) for an entire commercial.

- Switch to Classic Pushups (page 55) for as many commercials as you can.

- If you get tired, keep going with Knee Pushups (page 50).

Tip

When doing the "Cat" Stretch, don't lift your head to watch television while stretching. You'll just have to listen for a few seconds before relaxing in your chair.

- As your television program begins again, perform the "Cat" Stretch (page 31) before crawling back into that easy chair.

Commercial Break 6

- For one commercial, perform The "X" routine (page 57) before moving on to the rest of this break's exercises.

- For the remainder of the break, perform Elevated Triceps Pushups (page 62).

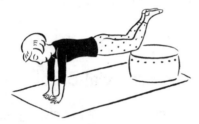

- Once your show begins again, be sure to stretch your Triceps (page 39) before settling back on the sofa.

Commercial Break 7

- Warm up with Sumo Squats (page 78) for one commercial.

- Start right into Progressive Reverse Lunges with a Slide Pulse (page 80) for the rest of the break. Switch legs for each commercial. Be sure to do some leg stretches as you settle back into your show.

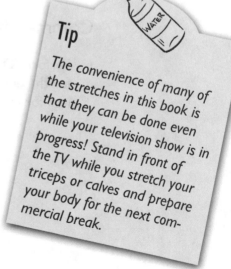

Tip

The convenience of many of the stretches in this book is that they can be done even while your television show is in progress! Stand in front of the TV while you stretch your triceps or calves and prepare your body for the next commercial break.

Commercial Break 8

Time for more legs! We can't forget those hamstrings.

* Do Hamstring Pulses (page 82) for an entire commercial break.

* Be sure to stretch the Hamstrings (page 35) when finished. If necessary, do this stretch during the first 30 seconds or so of your television show.

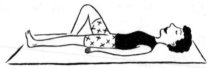

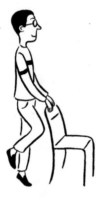

Commercial Break 9

* Do One-Legged Calf Raises (page 86). Switch legs with each new commercial.

* Again, be sure you stretch out those calves afterward!

Commercial Break 10

* Perform One-Legged Lunges (page 96) for the entire break, again switching legs for each new commercial.

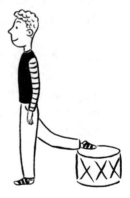

Commercial Break 11

It's crunch time! You should be familiar with the crunches in the book by now, so with each new product commercial, switch to a different crunch.

- Crunches (page 100)

- Elevated-Leg Crunches (page 101)

- Roll-Up Crunches (page 103)

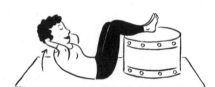

- Oblique Crunches (page 106)

- Bicycles (page 107)

- Crossover Crunches (page 108)

Commercial Break 12

Warm up your heart and lungs with one of the exercises from chapter 7. Start the exercise during the commercial and continue through your TV program.

- Marching in Place (page 123)

- Ice Skater's Move (page 124)

- Quick Steps (page 126)

Commercial Break 13

Cool down for this entire commercial break with some Marching in Place (page 123).

Final Commercial Break

Finish up with some stretching of any kind (see chapter 3) and Relaxed Breathing (page 20). You've earned it!

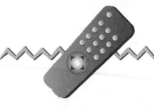

Program 6

If you've made it to this level, it is time to branch out. For example, instead of doing your balancing exercises while watching TV, try balancing on one leg while brushing your teeth or when waiting in line at the grocery store or bank. Practicing your balance while doing everyday things will help you progress in this very important area.

Commercial Break 1

*   Do the cardiovascular warm-up that works best for you (either Marching in Place [page 123] or the Ice Skater's Move [page 124]).

*   Follow this with some gentle stretches for the Chest (page 38), Reclining Neck Rolls (page 26), and the Upper Back and Shoulders (page 27). Do one stretch for each commercial.

Commercial Break 2

For each commercial, perform one of the following stretches:

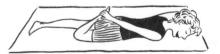

*   Hips and Butt (page 34)

*   Legs (page 35, 36, or 37)

Commercial Break 3

- For this commercial break, start with Classic Pushups (page 55). Perform as many pushups as you can for as many commercials as possible.

- If exhaustion or bad form sets in, switch to Knee Pushups (page 50).

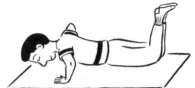

- Rest! You deserve it!

Commercial Break 4

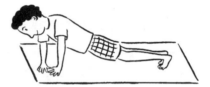

- Start with the Classic Triceps Pushups (page 64). If possible, try to get through the entire commercial break with this one exercise.

- If this gets too difficult, switch to The "X" (page 57).

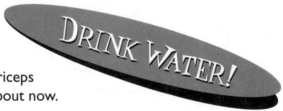

DRINK WATER!

- It's a good idea to do a Triceps stretch (page 39) right about now.

Commercial Break 5

It's time to work out your legs!

- Start your leg workout with Progressive Reverse Lunges with a Slide Pulse (page 80).

- If you make it through three rounds on each leg (one leg per commercial) and there are still more commercials, switch to the Sumo Squats (page 78) for the rest of the break.

Commercial Break 6

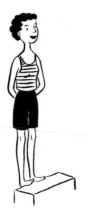

- Continuing with legs, get on the floor for Hamstring Pulses (page 82). Again, perform three rounds on each leg (one leg per commercial).

- If there are still more ads or if you get a particularly long commercial, finish the break working your calves by doing some Calf Raises with Changing Toe Positions (page 87).

Commercial Break 7

Let's mix this up a bit by combining Pulsing Lunges (page 73) with Step-Ups (page 77). Alternate legs, and exercises, with each commercial.

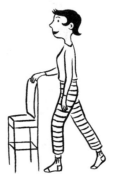

Commercial Break 8

Are your legs tired? If so, then crunches ought to be a welcome relief right about now. For each commercial, rotate to a different crunch.

- Crunches (page 100)

- Elevated-Leg Crunches (page 101)

- Roll-Up Crunches (page 103)

- Oblique Crunches (page 106)

- Bicycles (page 107)

- Crossover Crunches (page 108)

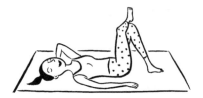

Commercial Break 9

The "guts" are finished; so it must be time for "butts"!

- Start with the most difficult exercise, One-Legged Lunges (page 96).

- If this becomes too exhausting, hit the floor and finish with some Reclining Butt Crushers (page 93).

Commercial Break 10

Enjoy this commercial break! You get to stretch the whole time. Pick out your favorites (you must have a few by now) and relax your muscles from head to toe. After stretching through the commercial break, get up and do your cardiovascular exercise for the next segment of the show. (Just because you are marching in place doesn't mean you can't watch TV at the same time!)

30-Minute Cardiovascular Interval

Use this pattern as you workout. Refer to the Borg Exertion Scale on page 120 for more information.

Commercial 1: 65% effort

Commercial 2: 75% effort

Commercial 3: 85% effort

Remaining Commercials: 55–60% effort

Commercial Break 11

- Cool down!

- Drink water!

- Pat yourself on the back!

Additional Challenges

Just when you thought it was safe to turn on your TV set . . . Here are some really challenging ideas to help you explore even more possibilities for you and your workout partner—the TV.

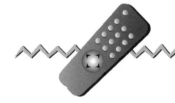

Circuit Workout for a 1-Hour TV program

In this exercise program, you'll use the commercials for muscle fitness and the TV show for cardiovascular fitness. It's total television fitness!

Before the Show Starts

Before you start the workout, be sure to warm up during the first commercial break and drink water.

- During the first commercial, pay close attention to your breathing and your posture. Look back to pages 12–13 for reminders on proper technique.

- For the second commercial, Marching in Place (page 123).

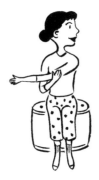

- For the remaining commercials, stretch the primary joints (Upper Back and Shoulders with a Twist [page 28], "Cat" Stretch [page 31], Hamstrings [page 35], Quadriceps [page 36], and Abdominals [page 40]).

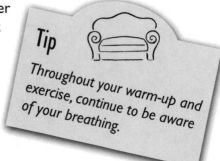

Tip

Throughout your warm-up and exercise, continue to be aware of your breathing.

Televion Program Part 1

- Sip your water and start to March in Place. Use your imagination. If there is music playing in the show, dance around for your marching in place. Or if you're watching something like "JAG," march along with the soldiers.

Commercial Break 1

- Do Chair Squats (page 70) for the first two commercials.

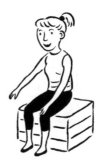

- For the next two commercials, do Pulsing Lunges (page 73) and alternate legs with each commercial.

- Move on to Sumo Squats (page 78) for the remaining commercials.

Back to the Show

It's boogie time! Get moving, but keep an eye on your exertion level. March in place; skate around the room. Whatever you do, just keep moving!

Commercial Break 2

- For the first two commercials, do Step-Ups (page 77).

- Next do some Pulsing Lunges (page 73). Perform the first set with the right leg forward. When the commercial changes, put the left leg forward.

- For the remaining commercials, do Reclining Butt Crushers (page 93).

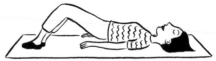

Back to the Show

Be sure to drink plenty of water as you do your cardiovascular workout.

Commercial Break 3

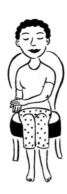

- Start with Classic Pushups (page 55) for two commercials.

- Proceed to Single-Arm Triceps Pushups (page 61) for the next two commercials. Alternate arms with each new commercial.

- Finish up the commercial break with Isometric Biceps Curls (page 67). Alternate arms with each new commercial.

Back to the Show

This is the final push! Stay hydrated and watch that exertion level . . . and have fun, of course!

Commercial Break 4

Perform the following exercises for two commercials each:

• Elevated-Leg Crunches (page 101)

• Roll-Up Crunches (page 103)

• Bicycles (page 107)

The Big Finale

Cool down with some gentle body movements and slow stretches. Great job!

30-Minute "Sit-Com" Circuit

This is similar to the 1-Hour Program set. Use the commercial breaks to do the exercises. Use the television show to get the heart pumping!

Television Show's Opening Vignette

• March or dance in place while you sing along with the show's theme song.

Commercial Break 1

Do one exercise per commercial.

• Pulsing Lunges (page 73)

• Sumo Squats (page 78)

Tip

So all you do is watch HBO? Don't let that stop you. While watching your favorite show or movie, alternate between 2 minutes of muscle fitness and 5 minutes of strengthening and 5 minutes of cardio work. But make sure you don't crane your neck just to see what's going on!

- One-Legged Butt Crushers (page 95)

- Elevated Pushups (page 52)

Back to the Show

Keep moving those legs and arms and keep that heart pumping!

Commercial Break 2

Again, do one exercise per commercial.

- Elevated Tricep Pushups (page 62)

- The "X" (page 57)

- Any abdominal exercise: Bicycles, Oblique Crunches, Challenging Crunches, Elevated-Leg Crunches (pages 100–110).

During the Closing Credits

Cool down and stretch. And drink lots of water.

Quickies

Here are some great exercise plans for when you have a few minutes—for instance, while waiting for something to print off the computer, for a program to download, or for your teenager to get off the phone. You get the idea! If you can accumulate 30 minutes of moderate physical activity per day, your health will be positively affected. Here are three "10-Minute Tune-Ups" to get you going . . . all you need is a clock or watch and a positive attitude.

Tune-Up 1

- Warm up by marching in place or dancing for 2 minutes

- Do each of these exercises/activities for 2 minutes: Crunches (page 100); Chair Squats (page 70); your favorite pushups (pages 46–56); and stretches for the upper back, legs, or chest (pages 27–29, 35–37, 38).

Tune-Up 2

- Warm up by doing the Ice Skater's Move for 1 minute.

- Do each of these exercises for 2 minutes: your favorite abdominals (pages 100–110), Hamstring Pulses (page 82), Triceps Wall Pushups (page 59), and the "Superman" back exercise (page 58).

- Cool down by stretching the lower back, neck, and legs for 1 minute.

Tune-Up 3

- Warm up for 2 minutes with Step-Ups (page 77).

- Alternate abdominal crunches with cardiovascular for 8 minutes (try alternating between 2 minutes of each).

We hope this chapter gives you an idea of how you can incorporate exercise and stretching into your everyday TV viewing activities. Don't let us limit you! Try some of your own combinations. Or if you outgrow this chapter, read on. Chapter 9 talks about different exercise equipment you can use to supplement your Commercial Break Workout.

9

What's Behind Door Number Two?

By now you have seen the value of taking an active role in improving your health and lifestyle habits. It is our hope that you will continue to use *The Commercial Break Workout* by adopting the F.I.T.T.R. (pronounced "Fitter") Principle. This is a clever fitness-industry acronym for:

Frequency: Exercise three times a week or more.

Intensity: Exercise the heart muscle at 50 percent to 85 percent of your maximum heart rate during your cardiovascular exercise and/or muscle fitness (as explained in chapter 7).

Time: Accumulate at least 30 minutes of exercise most days of the week.

Type: Vary the type of exercise to ensure retention and success, not to mention the fun factor.

Resistance: Engage in muscle fitness at least twice a week. Discover alternatives to improve the strength of your muscles.

The human body is designed to move. In fact, our bodies need to move. Just as we need water every day to survive, we also need a variety of movement to stay vital and healthy. Our brains control our movement. Therefore, if we are stingy with our energy expenditure, not only does our body suffer (muscles, tendons, ligaments, organs), but our brain suffers as well.

It is easy to fall into an exercise routine in which we do the same exercises, the same way, over and over. Repetition eventually teaches the body a pattern to which the brain readily conforms. This sort of patterning can lead to complacency, which, over time, increases physical degeneration. This means the body actually becomes resistant to change! When this happens, we set ourselves up for injury or some other uncomfortable dysfunction.

Believe it or not, muscles have "memory." If the exerciser repeats the same routine day in and day out, that exercise or exercise routine actually becomes less effective. By adding variety to workouts, therefore, we not only keep the workouts fresher and more interesting, but we also increase our fitness level and reduce our chances of injury.

Variety of movement and activity keeps the brain on its "toes." Exercise variety incorporates more muscles and, therefore, increases our brain activity. Ultimately, this all helps us become (or remain) functional and mobile. Therefore, no matter what ordinary chores and tasks we do throughout the day, we will be able to perform them with minimal strains, twitches, or twinges.

Another benefit to all of this variety of movement is the increased energy expenditure, or calorie burning (remember the "human furnace" discussion in chapter 1?). The more diverse our activities, the more muscle and brain matter we engage, the more the metabolism increases, the more calories our body burns, and the healthier we become.

The Commercial Break Workout presents plenty of options designed to stimulate your brain, engage your body, and keep you "tuned in" to fitness. As we all know, staying interested in exercise is half the battle!

Although *The Commercial Break Workout* is designed to help you get fit without the use of any equipment, other than your trusty television and a chair or two, you may eventually get bored and want to add to your regimen. Because variety is the key to keeping a body strong and healthy, we thought it fitting to suggest a few equipment alternatives just to help you keep things interesting. The following table introduces some fine, inexpensive fitness products that can help keep your mind and muscles nimble. Read on to obtain information on how to spice up your TV workouts.

The chart is followed by additional information from the manufacturers of each product.

Product	Primary Purpose/ Best Use	Manufacturer/ Description	Cost	Contact
FITBALL®	Cardiovascular, balance, flexibility, strength	Ball Dynamics (stability ball)	Approx. $30.00	800-752-2255 www.fitball.com
XERTUBES®	Strength, flexibility	SPRI Products (resistance tubes)	Approx. $7.00 each	800-222-7774 847-680-7550 (fax) www.spriproducts.com
AEROMAT®	Strength, flexibility, balance, stability	Found in the Power Systems catalog	Approx. $39.00	800-321-6975 www.power-systems.com
HYDRO-FIT®	Cardiovascular, strength	Hydro-Fit Wave Web® Pro (Hand mitts to add re- sistance in water)	Approx. $20.00	800-346-7295 www.hydrofit.com
HEART RATE MONITOR	Cardiovascular	Creative Health Products	$59–$99	800-742-4478 www.chponline.com www.scantechmedical.com
NEW LIFESTYLES DIGI- WALKER™	Cardiovascular	New Lifestyles	$27.00– $35.00	888-748-5377 www.digiwalker.com www.new-lifestyles.com

Ball Dynamics International, Incorporated

BALL DYNAMICS INTERNATIONAL, Incorporated has been promoting fitness products and educational materials from their Colorado location for more than 10 years. Among other things, the company offers an extended selection of high-quality Swiss balls, trademarked as FITBALL® exercise balls.

The Swiss ball was developed in Switzerland (yes, it really is Swiss!) in 1965 as a rehabilitation tool for children with cerebral palsy. Physical therapists discovered that by sitting on a round object, balance and reflex responses would improve more quickly. Swiss therapists approached an Italian toy manufacturer to start producing toy balls made of a more durable vinyl instead of rubber. The use of the ball quickly spread throughout Europe and is now widely accepted by physical therapists everywhere. The Fitball program most widely used in the United States was designed by Joanne Mayer, P.T., and Lindsay Zappala, B.A., to promote fun, safe, and effective exercise and rehabilitation programs that improve coordination, balance, flexibility, strength, faster reaction time, and even cardiovascular health. (The Fitball is fun to sit and bounce on like a trampoline!)

Today, the Fitball is used not only for therapy but also for general exercise and health improvement in all populations.

The Fitball is available in assorted shapes, sizes, and colors to accommodate just about every age, height, and ability level (and room decor!). It is an inexpensive tool and can be used in small spaces. You can even keep it in the living room.

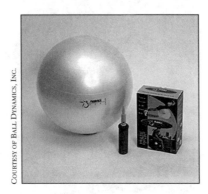

COURTESY OF BALL DYNAMICS, INC.

Instead of doing Marching in Place or the Ice Skater's Move for cardiovascular work, you can bounce up and down on your Fitball while watching TV. Or you can use it in place of balancing exercises.

SPRI Products, Incorporated

SPRI Products, Incorporated, is the leading manufacturer and distributor of rubberized resistance exercise products for the health and fitness industry. SPRI pioneered the use of rubber tubes as a simple, portable, easy-to-use method for strength training and building lean muscle tissue. It is the corporate objective of SPRI to remain state-of-the-art with consumers, providing convenient, affordable, effective, quality resistance exercise products.

The high-quality latex, Tough Tube™ XERTUBES® come in a variety of thicknesses and resistances and are equipped with sturdy, comfortable handles for ease of use. They are easy to pack into suitcases or to use in small spaces. Xertubes are versatile and effective for building muscle, enhancing general strength, and

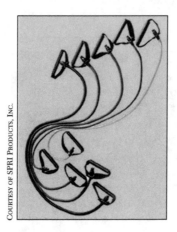

COURTESY OF SPRI PRODUCTS, INC.

improving flexibility. Because the tubes can be used in place of bulkier hand weights, people of all ages and fitness levels can use this product.

If you are getting bored with the weight-free biceps or triceps curls used in this book, use the Xertube to help out. Be sure to follow the instruction manual to ensure proper form. Then replace the exercises suggested in this book with some new exercises of your own!

You can obtain more information about the Xertube and shop online by visiting www.spriproducts.com.

Aeromat

The AEROMAT® is beautiful in its simplicity and is truly one of the most effective tools available for comfortably improving balance, ankle stability, strength, stamina, and coordination. Offered in the Power Systems catalog, the mat is made from smooth, soft, closed-cell foam that does not absorb water. It can be used while you work up a sweat without fear! The pad measures 19" × 16" × 2¹/2" and weighs only 2 pounds.

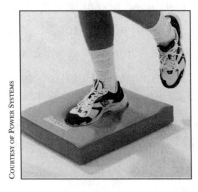

COURTESY OF POWER SYSTEMS

The Aeromat fits nicely with *ju* because it can be used with just about every exercise in the book. Simply by standing on this mat, you can turn even the easiest workouts into exercise routines that involve the core muscles of the back, gluteus, and abdomen! Use the Aeromat for posture and balance exercises, lunges, marching in place, and much more.

Many fine products are available from the Power Systems catalog. Peruse the whole catalog to find more ideas on how to tweak your exercise routines.

Hydro-Fit Corporation

HYDRO-FIT® Corporation makes quality products and accessories for use in the water. We are including a water exercise product because water is the perfect low-impact, supportive environment for a very effective workout. Because water is eight times denser than air, it is a great place to improve strength, cardiovascular health, and flexibility. And in the hot summer months, you can stay cool in the process! A water environment is effective because it supports the joints by the buoyancy effect on the body and because the water's density itself becomes a resistance tool.

Although many people enjoy water fitness for its own sake, Hydro-Fit has developed some fun, comfortable, effective products to enhance your experience and to create an even better workout. Even if all you like to do is stand in the water, you can get a fabulous workout with any of Hydro-Fit's products!

One particularly handy product from Hydro-Fit is a pair of gloves called WAVE WEB® PRO. These are comfortable,

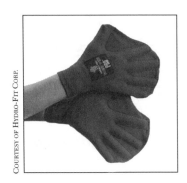

COURTESY OF HYDRO-FIT CORP.

durable gloves that turn your hands into ducklike webbed paddles! The gloves are constructed to allow water to actually pass through the material. This not only protects joints but also creates enough added resistance for a variable resistance workout. If you use the Wave Web Pro, start out by moving your hands through the water without the gloves. This will be your warmup. Once you are warmed up, add the Wave Web Pro and you'll see how much harder it is to move your hands through the water. This variation in the resistance will help your muscles get stronger. Using this product will also help improve cardiac output, enhance body strength, and support joint flexibility.

The affordable Wave Web Pro gloves are made of materials that can withstand the chemicals in pool water. So, take a TV break and splash around with this product! It comes in several sizes so the kids can enjoy them, too.

Heart Rate Monitors

If you are serious about reducing body fat, a heart rate monitor is one of the handiest products to own. Rather than relying on the Borg Exertion Scale (effective as it may be), you can use a heart rate monitor to find out just how hard you heart muscle is working. Let's face it, it is easy to go on a stroll and assume you have done an effective job for your cardiovascular system. But by using a heart rate monitor, you will be able to see exactly how effective that walk was. The monitor can even tell you when you are pushing yourself too hard.

To get the most out of your workout, you should frequently monitor your exercise intensity. Doing so will insure not only that you are working at a level that is safe for your age and ability but also that you are getting the most out of each workout. For example, if you work too intensely, you may injure yourself. If you're not working hard enough, however, you may get frustrated if you don't see expected results. Therefore we suggest using a heart rate monitor from the manufacturer of your choice to abet your success.

In addition to displaying your heart rate, heart rate monitors come with all sorts of features. Some of the more inexpensive ones include a night light and clock. While the more expensive ones may include a stop watch, calorie estimator, target zone alarms, date, safety-range warning alarms, and even software to

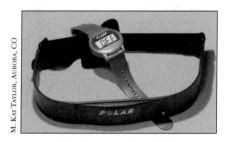

M. KAY TAYLOR, AURORA, CO

download data into your computer. One feature to consider when deciding which heart rate monitor to purchase is the safety-range warning alarm. This feature is particularly handy because, as we mature, our maximum heart rate decreases. This is not because our heartbeats get weaker as we age but because it takes longer for the heart to relax. In other words, it takes a bit longer for the heart to get ready for the next contraction. With this information, researchers have devised recommended beats per minute (BPM) for exercisers that correlate with their age group. When you enter your age into the heart monitor, you can choose the level of exertion you wish to achieve. The warning alarm will let you know if you are pushing too hard. This is important for people who have strict exercise guidelines, who are recovering from an illness in which cardiac heart rate needs to be watched, or who are new to exercise and are not yet comfortable judging how hard is too hard.

A heart rate monitor can look complex and intimidating but in fact it is very simple to use. Two pieces are involved: a strap to go around your chest and a watchlike device for your wrist, bicycle, or treadmill. The chest strap has a sensor that reads your heart rate. The sensor sends the information to the "watch" so you can read it digitally. Cool, huh!

There are many great heart rate monitor products to choose from. The most well-known company is POLAR®, which has several excellent models that cost less than $99.99. Other great companies with excellent models under $99.00 include CARDIO-SPORT® (www.cardiosport.com), ACUMEN® (www.acumen inc.com, 1-800-852-7823), REEBOK® (www.reebok.com), and LIFESOURCE® (www.lifesourceon line.com).

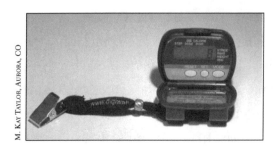

M. KAY TAYLOR, AURORA, CO

New Lifestyles

Activity burns calories. But how can you tell if you are moving enough? Since 1992, the folks at New Lifestyles have led the charge in finding simple ways for people to observe their own activity levels. The company has developed a simple to use, accurate pedometer called a DIGI-WALKER™. With its patented SECURITY STRAP™ (which has saved many a Digi-Walker from being flushed down a toilet!) and accurate and reliable sensor mechanism, the Digi-Walker is one of the best tools available for measuring how many steps you take in a day.

It is estimated by many medical and fitness professionals that if a person takes 10,000 steps a day, they will have walked about 4 or 5 miles. This would burn about 2,000 to 3,500 extra calories a week! Regardless of whether your goal is to lose weight or just become more fit, the Digi-Walker will show you that every step counts toward a fitter, leaner you.

Where Else Can I Go from Here?

In addition to the products mentioned above, there are plenty of other ways to expand your world of fitness. We know this is a radical thought, but get away from the glowing light of the TV set for a while. You don't need to join a fancy gym or buy expensive equipment. In fact, some of the best exercises out there are available almost for free. We say "almost" because, first of all, you need to buy this book! The second factor is appropriate clothing and other necessary gear. However, don't think you can use the "It costs too much" excuse (not that you would, of course!). Most of the activities we recommend in the rest of this chapter come pretty cheaply. So consider the following activities as possible supplements to your TV workouts.

Walking

It just may be your patriotic duty to start walking every day. Study after study has shown that the simple exercise of walking is very powerful medicine for warding off heart disease, a major medical expense not only to the consumer but also to insurance companies. If everyone in America would walk 20 to 30 minutes every day, our health-care bills could drop dramatically!

The only expenses you really incur for walking involve clothing: You want shoes that fit and that are designed for walking, and you want to wear weather-appropriate clothing. Good walking shoes are shaped so that the foot travels smoothly over the surface, keeping the toes from slapping down onto the ground. They are also lightweight and have a nice, wide toe box.

Another great tool to enhance your walking fun, and to help you burn more calories, is a pair of walking poles. They look like ski poles but are designed for pavement and trails. Using poles helps keep your upper body involved, which can boost your caloric output from 15 percent to 20 percent. And don't forget to wear your Digi-Walker!

Once you have done some aerobic shopping at your favorite mall (which is a fabulous place to walk, by the way—no bugs, rain, heat, or doggie detritus), you are ready to begin. Before heading out, think about safety. Because it's true that there is safety in numbers, get some of your friends together for a walk to discuss your favorite TV shows. If you have a dog, sign him up for your exercise program! Always carry a flashlight and a whistle, and wear something reflective so that drivers can see you.

Tip
To keep your walks even more interesting, use your walking log to record your thoughts while you walked or to note a funny or poignant instance along the way.

Start your program by choosing familiar ground that is relatively flat. It is also a good idea to wear a watch so you can time yourself on the decided-upon course. Keep a log describing how far you walked each day and record your time. You can even record your different routes, including notes on the terrain, time of day, and so forth. This way you will see your progress more readily and stay encouraged.

Time to get moving! If you are new to fitness walking, 15 to 20 minutes of walking is a good place to start. After about 7 minutes of an easy, gentle pace, stop and do some stretches (refer back to chapter 3). After about a minute or two of stretching, you are ready to pick up the pace.

Walking is not just a leg exercise. Your arms are involved as well. Keep your elbows bent at a 90-degree angle, stand up straight, squeeze your shoulder blades back and don't hunch your shoulders, and keep your arm movements swinging in a smooth, powerful arc. Believe it or not, using the arms correctly can boost your caloric burn by as much as 20 percent (according to Walk Off Weight newsletter, June 1997).

Keep your head up, chest up, and shoulders back. In a 1998 fitness handout, the IDEA Health and Fitness source suggested imagining someone dumping ice down your back to get the right mental picture of good walking posture . . . without the shivering. Smile and have some fun! Cool down for the last couple of minutes of your walk, being cognizant at all times of your perceived exertion levels.

Consistency is the key to any success, even walking. Put a gold star on the calendar or put a dollar in a jar for each day you do your walk. You will be amazed at how much better you feel after only a month of your walking program. If you find this activity to your liking, look for walking and hiking clubs (or start one of your own) in your town or neighborhood. That way you will always have company, conversation, and encouragement.

Swimming

Swimming is one of the greatest exercises you can do for yourself because it enables you to move your limbs through complete ranges of motion while being supported by water. The support of the water reduces the jarring and pounding on the joints often experienced by runners and walkers. The problem with swimming is that you need a pool. Fortunately, most communities have one or two public-access swimming pools where people can go for a nominal fee. Swimsuits are affordable, especially when purchased in the "off" season, and most of the other items some people use to make swimming more comfortable (swim caps, ear plugs, water shoes) can be purchased at discount sporting stores.

Because swimming involves all of the major muscle groups—legs, chest, back, shoulders, arms, and abdominals—it is a superior way to build muscle and burn fat.

If doing laps in the pool does not interest you, give water fitness classes a try. These classes offer one of the best ways to get a great workout without stressing the joints, jarring the spine, or sweating out your T-shirts. Water creates resistance in all directions. The harder you push, the more resistance you feel. Simply walking in water strengthens the legs and abdominal muscles, so imagine the benefits you will get in a class where you push, pull, twist, and "jog" in a gravity-free environment! All populations can benefit from this medium—disabled, injured, exercise beginners, elite athletes, young, old—and have a great time, too. Another great bonus is that you do not have to be a strong swimmer or even know how to swim to participate in most of the classes, because a vast majority of them are conducted while standing in the shallow end. You can have fun, stay cool, and feel fabulous.

Aquatic Fitness

According to the Aquatic Exercise Association, Inc., (AEA) aquatic fitness is defined as activities performed in the water that promote and enhance physical and mental fitness. It is typically performed in a vertical position in shallow and/or deep water. There are numerous applications to appeal to a wide variety of participants.

Water's unique properties allow the pool to provide an environment for people of all abilities. Buoyancy creates a reduced-impact exercise alternative that is easy on the joints, while the water's resistance challenges the muscles. Water lends itself to a well-balanced workout that improves all major components of physical fitness—aerobic training, muscular strength and endurance, flexibility, and body composition.

In the water, your body is buoyant and the impact to the joints during exercise is significantly less than on land. Depending on the water's depth, your body "weight" is reduced in the pool due to lessened gravitational forces.

- A body immersed to the neck bears approximately 10 percent of its body weight.

- A body immersed to the chest bears approximately 20 to 25 percent of its body weight.

- A body immersed to the waist bears approximately 50 percent of its body weight

A properly designed program in the water provides a highly effective workout in a safe and gentle environment. Shallow water programs are generally best performed in water that is about mid-chest depth for maximum comfort, control of movement, and optimum toning benefits for the upper body.

As we've mentioned in this book, muscles must work against resistance to become developed and toned. Water provides at least twelve times more resistance than air, which means that each movement in the pool is more challenging to the muscles. Also, muscles typically work in pairs. No matter which way you move your body or limbs through the water, you are always encountering resistance. This helps to provide a more balanced workout because opposing muscles are involved, unlike on land where you typically need to reposition the body or select a separate exercise to provide adequate stimulation to both muscles.

Finally, water cools more efficiently than air, so when exercising in the water, your body is able to eliminate excess heat more effectively. This is not to say that you will not sweat during a workout in the pool. Rather, water will help prevent overheating and washes away the perspiration as you exercise. Because water cools the body quickly, it is imperative that you begin every workout with a "thermal warm-up," which is designed to elevate the body's core temperature, warm the muscles, and prepare the joints for the increased workload to come.

Keep Those Doggies Rollin'!

Bicycling and rollerblading are two popular activities that provide a great workout while you speed over the ground. Expense can be a deterrent with these activities because the equipment is specialized to you, the participant. Bicycles need to be purchased and then fitted to your body type and fitness level. A helmet is an absolute must ("this is your head . . . this is your head on the pavement at 12 miles per hour . . ."), as are appropriate shoes for pedaling.

Rollerblading has similar concerns. Skates should be properly fitted by someone in the know, and wrist, elbow, and knee pads (helmets, too) should also be worn. Also, while bicycles can be ridden in plenty of areas (mountain bikes can go on trails; road bikes are great for highways; hybrids are terrific for paved trails), rollerblading needs a smooth, flat surface, especially for beginners. A few lessons on how to start, blade, and—especially—stop come in handy, as well!

Regardless of what you chose to do, by all means do what you love, or at least like. Don't get involved in activities that bore you to tears just because it is the latest cool thing. Use your imagination and keep your ears open for fun activities: dancing, fencing, karate, kickboxing, belly dancing—they are all out there waiting for you to discover them.

chapter ten

Wheel of (Food) Fortune

How to Survive the Days of Our Lives

D on't dig your grave with your own knife and fork" is an old English proverb, proving that culinary overindulgence is hardly a modern anomaly. However, never in our history have so many people weighed so much. A recent poll indicates that 80 percent of people over age twenty-five are overweight based on body mass index (BMI—a national guideline computed through a combination of weight and height). According to CNN.com, this figure has risen steadily, from 71 percent in 1995, 64 percent in 1990, and 58 percent in 1983. A report from Surgeon General David Satcher says that obesity is reaching "epidemic proportions" and could soon cause as much preventable disease and death as does smoking. According to Dr. Satcher, the condition of being overweight or obese causes as many as 300,000 premature deaths each year. The Centers for Disease Control and Prevention has written in the *Journal of the American Medical Association*, "Clearly, genes related to obesity are *not* responsible for the epidemic of obesity because the U.S. gene pool did not change significantly between 1991 and 1999."

The United States is one of the few countries in the world where the majority of its citizens have the luxury of choosing not only the type of food they eat but also the frequency at which they eat it. Food and beverage companies spend *billions* of dollars annually to influence decisions in both of those arenas. The sideshow in this mad scramble for your attention (and your money) is the fruit and vegetable industry, which is lucky if it can manage a few *million* dollars to get your attention. With the advertising scales tipped aggressively toward the large snack-food production companies and fast-food restaurants, the choices we make are often done without the best available information. The purpose of this chapter is to provide facts and useful information so you can choose wisely.

The Basics

- A calorie is a measure of energy. Our bodies require a certain number of calories to keep us healthy and alive. Food = Fuel for humans, just as Gas = Fuel for cars.

- Calories count ... *all* of them, even the "fat-free" calories.

- Carbohydrates (complex carbohydrates = fruits, vegetables, whole grains, beans/legumes, sweet potatoes, yams; simple carbohydrates = sugars, starches [like white potatoes or pasta], and processed grains) and proteins (meat, fish, dairy) are calculated at 4 calories per gram. Fats (butters, oils) are calculated at 9 calories per gram. Alcohol is worth 7 calories per gram.

- Any excess calories that are not used are stored primarily in our insatiable fat cells.

- I pound of fat = 3,500 calories. Therefore, if you reduce your daily intake of food by 250 calories *and* add a daily activity that burns 250 calories per day, you could lose about one pound per week.

- It is *never* healthy to eat fewer than 1,200 calories per day.

- *Eat breakfast.* After sleeping for 6 to 8 hours, your body's metabolism (the rate at which your body burns calories) needs to be "jump-started." It is recommended that you eat a meal containing complex carbohydrates (fruit, vegetables, whole grains) and some protein (skim milk, yogurt, cottage cheese). Whole grain cereals such as Shredded Wheat, Grape-Nuts, and Muselix are better than Cocoa Puffs, Cap'n Crunch, and other cereals high in sugar and low in fiber. Oh, and please remember, a muffin is just a cupcake without the icing. You can do better . . .

- A healthy lunch will include about 3 ounces (about the size of a deck of cards) of protein along with vegetables and whole grains. This will keep you from falling asleep at your desk at 2:00 P.M.!

- Make dinner the lightest meal of the day. It's no fun going to bed hungry, and it's unhealthy going to bed full. How to hit the right balance? Eat small snacks of about 250 calories every 2 1/2 to 3 hours during the day. Try fruit, yogurt, lowfat cheese and whole grain crackers, or vegetables with a lowfat dipping sauce.

- Size matters! Portions that is . . . Watch out for the portion sizes on the foods that you order or serve to yourself. An article in the *Denver Post* suggests that you use your hand as a measuring tool: your palm = 3 ounces; a fist = 1 cup; a handful = 1–2 ounces of snack food; a thumb = 1 ounce of cheese.

Helpful Tips for Healthful Shopping

Watching TV can lead to a lot of mindless eating, which can easily pack in hundreds of unwanted calories. However, snacking is part of the TV culture. What to do? A good place to make changes is at the grocery store. Try some of these ideas:

- Always make a *list* when you go to the grocery store . . . and stick to it!

- *Never* shop for food when you are hungry. Eat something first.

- Remind yourself that "fat-free" and "cholesterol-free" do not mean "calorie-free." Sometimes the caloric difference between the regular cookie and the one that is fat-free is minimal. Why? Fat carries flavor. Without fat, sugar becomes a more important ingredient.

- Have a *plan!* If you jot down specific meal and snack ideas ahead of time, it's less likely that you'll be capricious with your caloric allowance.

- Keep a personal *food diary* of your daily diet. This way you will become familiar with the calorie counts of your favorite foods and you can shop (and eat) accordingly.

Basic Guidelines for Good Nutrition

Humans need a variety of foods to achieve optimum health. Remember the "Four Basic Food Groups" (meats, dairy, fruits and vegetables, and grains) you learned about in elementary school? They're baaaaaaack! Only now they've been divided into Five Basic Food Groups: vegetables, fruits, grains, meats, and milk. Please note that there is still no Donut and Chocolate Food Group. It is a good idea to try a variety of foods within each group, so that (a) you are sure to get all of the nutrients that you need each day, and (b) you don't get bored to death with your food. The more physically active you are, the more calories you will need. Experiment with various eating plans and quantities until you find your own personal niche and comfort level.

Nothing separates a vulnerable person from his money faster than a "guaranteed miracle weight-loss plan." Rather than wasting time, money, hopes, and dreams on these alleged "sure-fire shortcuts," we highly recommend the services of a registered dietitian to help you sort through your personal caloric and nutritional needs. Education is power. Become educated through reliable sources.

Hits and Myths:
Red Flags, Fallacies, and Facts

Exercise creates muscle; *diet* exposes it. We are using the word "diet" only as it applies to a healthful food regimen. In other words, we promote and encourage the sensible eating of a variety of foods. We do *not* support the concept of "diet" as the word is used by the weight-loss industry, in which you are told to restrict yourself to certain foods or combinations of foods. "Dieting," being "on a diet," and so forth are usually self-defeating practices. Remember, if it sounds too good to be true, it is. If "rapid weight loss" is promised, be aware that such a thing is both unlikely and unhealthful.

The following are some of the more popular food myths, along with a reasonable accounting of the truth.

MYTH #1.   *"Carbohydrates make you fat, and high-protein diets make fat melt away."*

FACT. "Fat burns in the flame of carbohydrate," says Daniel Kosich, exercise science co-editor for *Shape* magazine. Fruits, vegetables, whole grains, and beans are nutritionally dense complex carbohydrates that are not only essential for good health but also necessary for proper fat utilization. Highly processed foods—such as crackers, chips, cookies, and some breads—are often loaded with sugar and fat, high in calories, and nutritionally empty. Eating a small amount of protein (about the size of the palm of your hand) three times a day is all most people need for good health.

Any food will be stored as fat when more calories are consumed than the body needs, regardless of whether the calories are carbohydrates, proteins, or fats. Many promoted "diets" work, not because of magic combinations or the elimination of certain foods, but because calories are restricted. By following any calorie-restricted plan, weight will be lost—period. High-protein diets are often too high in fat and can place an inordinate strain on the liver and kidneys.

MYTH #2. *"Water should always be consumed ice cold
because your body uses more calories to
heat it up."*

FACT. Water is best absorbed by the body at about room temperature. The notion that our body has to expend more calories
to warm the water is wishful thinking! While we're on the subject
of water, too much water at mealtime can interfere with digestion. An 8–10 ounce glass of water with meals is appropriate.
Remember that water contains zero calories. Sodas, juices, and
alcoholic beverages are much higher in calories than most people
realize. Take this into account when tracking your caloric intake.

MYTH #3. *"Caffeine, ephedra (ma huang), and ginseng
give you energy and boost metabolism."*

FACT. *Energy* comes from *calories*—period. Caffeine and other
herbal substances may give you a "buzz" and jangle your nerves,
but this is *not* energy. You can boost your metabolism by increas-
ing your body's lean muscle. Beware of any claim that a pill will
"melt away fat."

MYTH #4. *"To lose weight, all fat should be eliminated
from your diet."*

FACT. Fat is essential for good health. As with all foods, fats
must be balanced properly in a healthful diet. Saturated fats
(primarily from animals and coconut and palm oils) can end up
on the walls of your arteries. Unsaturated fats (primarily from
vegetables and grains) are much easier for the body to use.

Vitamins A, E, D, and K are all fat-soluble, meaning that fat is
needed for these necessary vitamins to be used properly by the

body. A healthful diet obtains about 20 to 25 percent of its total calories from fat, with only 10 percent from saturated sources.

MYTH #5.   "Never mix carbohydrates with proteins."

FACT. The strange notion that food combining is bad for the body seems to rear its head every decade. The human body was designed to break down many types of food at the same time. If nature did not intend for this to be healthful, why would milk (human and animal), legumes (such as peanuts), grains, and many other foods naturally contain both carbohydrates and proteins? Consuming a wide variety of whole foods in amounts appropriate for your particular body composition and lifestyle is what really matters.

MYTH #6.   "If I smoke, I will lose weight."

FACT. It is *always* a good idea to quit smoking. Some people may gain weight temporarily when they quit; others may not. According to the American Lung Association, any weight gain that results from quitting smoking should disappear once that highly addictive drug, nicotine, is out of the system. Many smokers lose weight simply because smoking takes the place of eating. However, tobacco is cured with sugar, and cigarette paper contains sugar, which can induce some powerful cravings for sweets and other high-calorie snacks. Either way, it's not exactly a healthy plan! Because smokers get used to a hand-to-mouth ritual, when they quit, they often feel the need to eat just to keep that hand going toward the mouth.

Exercise to the rescue! If you quit smoking, use exercise and healthful eating to help restore your body to good health.

According to Max A. Schneider, M.D., chairman of the board of directors of the National Council on Alcoholism and Drug Abuse, exercise can lower cardiac-related death for smokers by up to 40 percent. Also, "the endorphins released through exercise help neutralize the cravings and combat the depression that most new nonsmokers face."

MYTH #7. "Never eat after 6:00 P.M."

FACT. Most nighttime eating is due to a relaxed atmosphere in the comfort of the home after a long day's work. The refrigerator is usually in proximity to the TV and lounge chair, and it offers one temptation after another. Digestion does tend to slow down at the end of the day, so eating late and going to bed on a full stomach is generally a bad idea. Ideally, there should be a 3-hour window between a large meal and bed. However, hunger happens, and so does insomnia. To stop the craving, it's perfectly acceptable to consume a small snack later in the evening, such as a piece of fruit, a small scoop of nuts, or a half-cup of cottage cheese. Stay away from sugar, however, as that can cause even more lack of sleep thanks to the sugar content!

MYTH #8. "Skipping meals is a good way to lose weight."

FACT. This is the method used by sumo wrestlers to *gain* weight! Sumo wrestlers skip breakfast, exercise on an empty stomach, eat a large meal in the late afternoon (followed by a nap), then eat another large meal late in the day before going to sleep. Dr. James Hill, an obesity researcher at the University of Colorado Health Sciences Center, has found that the body actually adapts to this pattern of eating by learning not only to expect a large delivery of food but also how to store it quickly.

Many people complain that they are simply not hungry in the morning or that they don't have time to eat lunch. Even if you think you're not hungry, try to eat a little something to retrain your body to want fuel on a more regular basis (unless, of course, you're training to be a sumo wrestler).

MYTH #9.   "Vinegar and grapefruit melt body fat."

FACT. Once again, *no* food instantly melts away body fat. The acidic taste of both vinegar and grapefruit can temporarily stop you from wanting more food, but scientifically, there is no evidence that these foods have magic thermodynamic properties.

MYTH #10. "Most people are fat because of genetics or a slow metabolism."

FACT. Wrong. Most people are fat because they eat too many calories compared with the number of calories they expend. Metabolism increases with the development of more lean muscle. Although there may be a genetic disposition to have more fat cells, regular exercise and a healthful caloric intake can fool Mother Nature!

Stay Tuned for Scenes from Next Week's Program . . .

You have completed the easiest, most practical "TV Guide" available for improved health for the avid television watcher. Enjoy the healthy changes, scream like Xena (yiyiyiyi!), and be a Survivor!

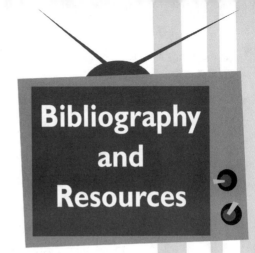

Bibliography and Resources

Books

Anderson, Bob. *Stretching*. Bolinas, CA: Shelter Publications, 1980.

Bailey, Covert. *Fit or Fat?* Boston: Houghton Mifflin, 1978.

Bailey, Covert. *Smart Exercise*. New York: Houghton Mifflin, 1984.

Berkow, Robert, M.D. (ed.). *The Merck Manual of Medical Information*. Whitehouse Station, NJ: Merck Research Laboratories, 1997.

Blakey, Paul. *The Muscle Book*. Honesdale, PA: Himalayan Institute Press, 1992.

Calais-Germain, Blandine. *Anatomy of Movement*. Seattle: Eastland Press, 1991.

Calais-Germain, Blandine, and Andre Lamotte. *Anatomy of Movement Exercises*. Seattle: Eastland Press, 1992.

Clark, Nancy, M.S., R.D. *Nutrition: Nancy Clark's Sports Nutrition Guidebook* (2nd edition). Champaign, IL: Human Kinetics, 1990.

Cotton, Richard T. (ed.). *Exercise for Older Adults* (American Council on Exercise). Champaign, IL: Human Kinetics, 1998.

Cotton, Richard T., and Ross E. Anderson (eds.). *Clinical Exercise Specialist Manual.* San Diego, CA: American Council on Exercise, 1999.

DeVries, Herbert A. *Physiology of Exercise for Physical Education and Athletics* (4th edition). Dubuque, IA: Wm C. Brown Publishers, 1986.

Dunne, Lavon J. *Nutrition Almanac* (3rd edition). New York: McGraw-Hill, 1990.

Floyd, R. T., and Clem Thompson. *Manual of Structural Kinesiology.* WCB/McGraw, 1998.

Heller, Joseph, and William A. Henkin. *Bodywise.* Oakland, CA: Wingbow Press, 1991.

Howley, Edward T., and B. Don Franks. *Health/Fitness Instructor's Handbook.* Champaign, IL: Human Kinetics, 1996.

Kosich, Daniel, Ph.D. *Get Real, A Personal Guide to Real-Life Weight Management.* San Diego, CA: IDEA, 1995.

Luttgens and Wells. *Kinesiology, Scientific Basis of Human Motion* (7th edition). CBS College Publishing.

Tkac, Debora (ed.) and Editors of *Prevention Magazine. Everyday Health Tips.* Emmaus, PA: Rodale Press, 1988.

Ulene, Art, M.D. *Take It Off! Keep It Off!* Berkeley, CA: Ulysses Press, 1995.

Van Gelder, Naneene (ed.). *Aerobic Dance-Exercise Instructor Manual.* IDEA Foundation, 1987.

Whitney, Eleanor, and Eve Hamilton. *Understanding Nutrition.* St. Paul, MN: West Publishing, 1987.

Yessis, Michael, Ph.D. *Kinesiology of Exercise.* Indianapolis, IN: Masters Press, 1992.

Magazine Articles, Newsletters, Professional Journals, and Reports

Arnold, Joan. "Move It or Lose It." *My Generation,* May–June 2001, p. 23.

Barone, Jeanine. "Five New Reasons to Get Physical." *Eating Well,* July/August 1995.

Bloor, James L. "Quit and Get Fit." *Prime Health & Fitness,* Summer 1998, p. 39.

Brody, Jane. "Had Enough Water to Drink? Probably Not." *Denver Post,* 17 June 1996, p. F1.

Clemens-Silence, Michele, M.A. "Exercises Buried Treasure." *IDEA Today,* 1995.

Cobb, Elissa. "Working with the Inactive." *IDEA Personal Trainer,* July/August 1995.

Costill, D. L. "Carbohydrates for Exercise: Dietary Demands for Optimal Performance." *International Journal of Sports Medicine* 9 (1988).

Cotton, Richard T. (ed.). *ACE Certified News* 4(2)–8(2), March 1998–March 2002.

Cotton, Richard T., M.A. *ACE Fitness Matters Series* 1–8, May 1995–February 2002.

"Could You Be More Active?" *Reebok Alliance Newsletter,* 1994.

Dunn Bates, Colleen. "Past Perfect." *Cooking Light,* June 1996.

Fenton, Mark. "Be Active." *The Walking Magazine,* May/June 1996.

"Fitness Facts: Blue Cross Blue Shield of Vermont, Healthwise Handbook" (13th edition), 1997, chapter 17.

"Food Power" (3rd edition), National Dairy Council, Rosemont, IL.

Francis, Lorna, Ph.D. "Setting Smart Goals." *IDEA Personal Trainer*, 1994.

"The Health Letter," XV(2), January 25, 1980.

Jacobson, Michael F., Ph.D. (executive director). *Nutrition Action Health Letter* 18(8)–29(2), October 1992–March 2002.

Kleiner, Susan. "A Few Facts on Fluids." *IDEA Today*, April 1995, p. 61.

Kravitz, Len, M.A., and Robert Robergs, Ph.D. "To Be Active or Not to Be Active?" *IDEA Today*, March 1993.

Kravitz, Len, M.A., and Robert Robergs, Ph.D. "Why Should I Exercise?" *IDEA Today*, 1993.

LaForge, Ralph, M.S. "Revised Exercise Standards." *IDEA Today*, May 1995.

Legwold, Gary. "Do a Little, Get a Lot." *Better Homes and Gardens*, September, 1995.

Margen, Sheldon, M.D. "A Myth That Never Dies." *UC Berkeley Wellness Letter* 17(3), p. 8.

Munson, Marty, with Michele Stanten. "Fat Proof Your Figure After 40." *Prevention*, April 1996.

Munson, Marty, with Sharon Stocker. "Make Exercise Automatic. Natural Weight Control." *Prevention*, January 1996.

Northrup, Christiane, M.D.. "How Your Breath Can Change Your Life." *Health for Women* 4(11): pp. 1–3, November 1997.

Nutrition Newsletters, Spring, Summer, Fall, Winter, 1998/1999.

Parker, Victoria. "Eight Ways to Stop Aging in its Tracks." *The Walking Magazine*, May/June 1996.

Pennebaker, Ruth. "Take Back Your Time." *Cooking Light*, 1995.

"Physical Fitness and All Cause Mortality, A Prospective Study of Healthy Men and Women," *The Journal of the American Medical Association* 262, 1989.

Roach, Mary. "The World's Biggest Weight Experts." *Health,* March–April 1993, pp. 62–72.

Robb-Nicholson, Celeste, M.D. (ed.) *Harvard Women's Health Watch* 3(1)–9(6), September 1995–February 2002.

Rosenson, Robert S., M.D. "New Cholesterol Guidelines." *Bottomline Health* 15(9): pp. 5–6, September 2001.

Satcher, David, M.D. Speech at the launch of "Healthy People 2010. Washington, DC, 24–28 January 2000.

Schlosberg, Suzanne. "How You Can Have Fit, Beautiful Legs?" *The Walking Magazine,* March/April 1996.

Schlosberg, Suzanne. "Look Good. Feel Good. Be Strong." *The Walking Magazine,* November/December 1995.

Schreiber, Kay, Med, CSCS. "I Just Don't Have Time!" *IDEA Personal Trainer,* November/December 1994.

Sheller, Robert, M.D. (ed.). "Weight Control, What Works and Why." *Mayo Clinic Health Letter Supplement,* 2001.

"Smart Heart Grocery List." Coors Wellness Center, Golden, CO, 1998.

Smith, Kerri. "Puzzled by Pounds?" *Denver Post,* 1 August 1999, F1, F10.

Sports Science Exchange 11(3 and 33), 1998; 9(3), 1998.

Staff. "Adding Muscle to the Diet." *IDEA Personal Trainer,* June 1996.

Staff. "Brief Walks Pay Off." *Cooking Light,* September 1997.

Staff. "Short Bouts Produce Big Results." *Health,* January/February 1999, p. 107.

Swartzberg, John Edward, M.D., F.A.C.P. (ed.). *University of California, Berkley Wellness Letter* 18(1)–18(8), December 2001–May 2002.

Teare, Tracy (ed.). "Walk Off Weight" (*Walking* magazine's weight-loss newsletter). 1(2)–2(6), January 1996–June 1997.

Westcott, Wayne, Ph.D. "Seven Up," *Men's Confidential,* December 1995.

Wood, Michael, PTA, CSCS. "Getting a Leg Up on Strength." *The Walking Magazine,* November/ December 1995.

Internet Web Sites

The Blonz Guide to Nutrition, Food Science, and Health: www.blonz.com

Center for Science in the Public Interest: www.cspinet.org

Centers for Disease Control and Prevention: www.cdc.gov

CNN.com—Health: www.cnn.com/HEALTH/

Dr. Koop: www.drkoop.com

End Sedentary Death Syndrome: www.ridinactivity.org

FitnessManagement.com: www.fitnessworld.com

The Food Doctor: Foods for Mind and Body: www.thefooddoctor.com

National Institute on Aging of the National Institutes of Health: www.nia.nih.gov

National Institute of Diabetes & Digestive & Kidney Diseases of the National Institutes of Health: www.niddk.nih.gov

Office of the Surgeon General: www.surgeongeneral.gov

Southwest Bariatric Nutrition Center: Dr. Donald S. Robertson: www.weight-control.com/doctor.html

WebMD: www.webmd.com

Index

About the Authors

Linda J. Buch, an ACE-certified personal fitness trainer, is also a weekly columnist for the Sunday *Denver Post* Lifestyles section, writing a question/answer fitness column called "Body Language" (trademark pending). She has spent most of her life involved in the field of fitness, both through personal participation and by teaching others. After receiving a Bachelor of Arts degree in health education and history, with a minor in physical education, from Wittenberg University, Springfield, Ohio, in 1972, she was hired by the Lancaster, Pennsylvania, YMCA to be their first Women's and Girls' Physical Activities Director. In that position, she was responsible for introducing programs such as coed aerobics, water fitness, and children's exercise.

Because travel has always been of great interest to Linda, she applied to and was hired by Continental Airlines, where she spent nine years as a flight attendant. During that time, she took advantage of every opportunity to see the world. After leaving the airlines in 1983, she returned to school, Chapman College, and began work on her Masters Degree in sports medicine. While working as the general manager for a gym in Denver, Linda became involved in bodybuilding and, after only one year of training, became a local champion, winning the Rocky Mountain Regional Open Championship. She was then invited to compete nationally at the Women's Championships in Miami in 1986. This experience encouraged her to compete only in competitions in which contestants were tested for steroids and other drugs. In 1990, due to her busy schedule as a personal fitness trainer, she gave up bodybuilding competition.

Since 1987, Linda has run her own personal training business, working individually with adults throughout the Denver Metro area.

Seth Anne Snider-Copley is a native Coloradan currently residing in Lyon, France, with her husband. She is an exercise physiologist and kinesiotherapist, nationally and internationally recognized for her knowledge and expertise in the fitness industry. She graduated with a Bachelor of Science degree from Miami University in 1989 and pursued graduate studies in occupational therapy at both the University of Illinois in Chicago and at the University of Colorado in Denver.

Her involvement in the fitness and wellness industry began in 1985, when she was selected to be a student-trainer for Division I football and soccer. After college graduation, she interned with the Coors Wellness Center in Golden, Colorado, specializing in gerontology and cardiac rehabilitation. After completing graduate studies in Chicago in 1991, she was hired as a Lifetime Skills Specialist at MENTOR, where she worked with a multidisciplinary team of paraprofessionals, designing programs to reintegrate medically complex individuals back into society. In 1992, Seth and another fitness professional formed Urban Fitness, Inc., a post-rehabilitative and personal training company in the Chicago area, where she had the opportunity to work as a strength training coach for nationally recognized ice skaters. She designed and implemented personal training programs to hundreds of clients. In addition, she was involved in founding a program for young children in one of Chicago's Cabrini Green elementary schools. The program offered "movement breaks" for children who had lost all extracurricular activities due to lack of city funding. After relocating back to Denver, Colorado, Seth was involved with yet another volunteer project and with writing a grant for the Southwestern Improvement Council (SWIC). The grant helped fund programs and activities for underprivileged families of various ethnic backgrounds. The programs helped educate the families on the topics of health and wellness

In 1993, Seth decided to pursue her own business, forming Fitness West, LLC. Seth is a well-known and respected aquatic specialist chosen by executive committee to represent the Aquatic Exercise Association (AEA) as an international presenter and chosen by Fitour as an international presenter and lecturer on post-rehabilitation and general fitness. She has worked with many elite and Olympic athletes during her seventeen years as a fitness specialist and kinesiotherapist. She is a continuing education provider for the American Council on Exercise (ACE), the AEA, and Aerobic Fitness Association of America (AFAA). Her certifications include the American Heart Association (CPR instructor), the American Red Cross (Water Safety Instructor), the Kenneth Cooper Institute for Aerobic Research (IAR), and the Aquatic Exercise Association (AEA).